The Basic Food & Brand-Name Calorie Counter

The Basic Food & Brand-Name Calorie Counter

(*Excerpted from "The Dictionary of Calories and Carbohydrates"*)

BARBARA KRAUS

Grosset & Dunlap
Publishers, New York

For Mon Ling, Karl and Ling Ling Landegger

INTRODUCTION

Most of the data presented here are derived from my book THE DICTIONARY OF CALORIES AND CARBOHYDRATES. In that book, 9,000 brand names and basic foods were listed with their calories and carbohydrate count.

In this smaller book I have made certain compromises: whereas in the giant book there were several physical descriptions, here there is but one; when there is only one calorie variation between products the products have been grouped together. (Such variations are unimportant and often are only the result of a different way of rounding numbers.) Finally, no dietetic products are included that are dietetic only because they are sodium restricted because the calories are not affected.

For you who have never before had an interest in weight control, I offer the following necessary information.

A Calorie

A calorie is a short hand way to summarize the units of energy contained in any foodstuff or alcoholic beverage, similar to the way a thermometer indicates heat. One pound of fat is equal to 3500 calories. Add this number of calories to those you need to balance your energy requirement and you will gain one pound; subtract it and you will lose a pound.

How To Use This Book

To begin with, you use this book like a dictionary. If your plan is to cut down on calories, the easiest way to do so is to consult the calorie counter and keep an accurate count of your total intake of food and beverages for a period of seven days. If you have not gained or lost weight during that week, divide that number by 7 and you'll have your maintenance diet expressed in calories. To lose weight, you must reduce your daily or weekly intake of calories below this maintenance level. To gain, increase the intake.

Keeping in mind that you want to stay healthy and eat well-balanced meals (which include the basic food groups: milk or milk products; meat, poultry or fish; vegetables and fruits; and whole grain or enriched breads or cereals, as well as some fats or oils), you then start to cut down on your portions in order to reduce your intake of calories. There are many imaginative ways to diet without total withdrawal from one's favorite foods. Once you know and don't have to guess what calories are in your foods, you can relax and enjoy them. It could turn out that dieting isn't so bad after all.

ABBREVIATIONS AND SYMBOLS

* = prepared as packaging directs[1]
< = less than
& = and
" = inch
canned = bottles or jars as well as cans
dia. = diameter
fl. = fluid
liq. = liquid
lb. = pound
med. = medium

oz. = ounce
pkg. = package
pt. = pint
qt. = quart
sq. = square
T. = tablespoon
Tr. = trace
tsp. = teaspoon
wt. = weight

Italics or name in parentheses = registered trademark, ®.
All data not identified by company or trademark are based upon material obtained from the United States Department of Agriculture.

EQUIVALENTS

By Weight

1 pound = 16 ounces
1 ounce = 28.35 grams
3.52 ounces = 100 grams

By Volume

1 quart = 4 cups
1 cup = 8 fluid ounces
1 cup = ½ pint
1 cup = 16 tablespoons
2 tablespoons = 1 fluid ounce
1 tablespoon = 3 teaspoons
1 pound butter = 4 sticks or 2 cups

[1]If the package directions call for whole or skim milk, the data given here are for whole milk, unless otherwise stated.

The Basic Food
& Brand-Name
Calorie
Counter

Food and Description	Measure or Quantity	Calories

A

ABALONE:
Raw, meat only	4 oz.	111
Canned	4 oz.	91

AC'CENT | ¼ tsp. | 3

ALMOND:
In shell	4 oz.	347
Shelled, whole	1 oz.	170
Blanched, slivered (Blue Diamond)	1 cup	1008
Flavored (Blue Diamond)	1 oz.	180
Roasted, diced (Blue Diamond)	1 oz.	176

ALPHA-BITS (Post) | 1 oz. | 113

AMBROSIA, chilled (Kraft) | 4 oz. | 85

ANCHOVY PASTE (Crosse & Blackwell) | 1 oz. | 40

ANCHOVY, PICKLED | 1 oz. | 50

ANGEL FOOD CAKE:
Loaf (Van de Kamp's)	10-oz. loaf	1006
Ring, chocolate-iced (Van de Kamp's)	7½" cake	2525

ANGEL FOOD CAKE MIX:
*(Betty Crocker):		
1 step	1 cake	1332
2 step	1 cake	1200
Confetti	1 cake	1368
Lemon custard	1 cake	1332
Strawberry	1 cake	1380
*(Duncan Hines)	1 cake	1572
(Pillsbury)	1 oz.	102
*(Swans Down)	1 cake	1584

*Prepared as Package Directs

Food and Description	Measure or Quantity	Calories
ANISE EXTRACT:		
(Ehlers)	1 tsp.	12
(French's)	1 tsp.	26
APPLE:		
Eaten with skin	1 lb.	242
Eaten without skin	1 lb.	211
Dehydrated, uncooked	1 oz.	100
Dried, uncooked (Del Monte)	1 cup	212
Frozen, sweetened, slices	4 oz.	105
APPLE BUTTER:		
(Bama)	1 T.	27
(Smucker's) spiced	1 T.	30
APPLE CIDER, cherry or sweet		
(Motts)	½ cup	59
APPLE DRINK:		
(Del Monte)	6 fl. oz.	84
(Hi-C)	6 fl. oz.	87
APPLE JACKS (Kellogg's)	1 oz.	112
APPLE JELLY:		
(White House)	1 T.	46
Low calorie (Slenderella)	1 T.	25
APPLE JUICE (Heinz)	5½-fl.-oz. can	88
APPLE PIE:		
(Drake's)	2-oz. pie	200
(Tastykake)	4-oz. pie	380
Frozen:		
(Banquet)	5-oz. serving	351
(Morton)	20-oz. pie	1440
(Morton)	24-oz. pie	1620
(Morton)	46-oz. pie	3096
(Mrs. Smith's)	8″ pie	1814
(Mrs. Smith's) natural juice	9″ pie	2888
(Mrs. Smith's)	10″ pie	3106
Dutch apple (Mrs. Smith's)	8″ pie	1856
Tart (Mrs. Smith's)	8″ pie	1501

*Prepared as Package Directs

Food and Description	Measure or Quantity	Calories
APPLE PIE FILLING:		
(Comstock)	½ cup	178
French (Comstock)	½ cup	97
(Lucky Leaf)	8 oz.	248
(Musselman's)	½ cup	142
Unsweetened (Lucky Leaf)	8 oz.	98
APPLESAUCE:		
Sweetened:		
(Del Monte)	½ cup	119
(Hunt's)	5-oz. can	94
(Seneca) cinnamon	½ cup	134
(Seneca) 100% McIntosh	½ cup	116
(Stokely-Van Camp)	½ cup	109
(White House)	½ cup	110
Unsweetened:		
(Blue Boy)	4 oz.	43
(Diet Delight)	½ cup	58
(Mott's)	½ cup	56
(S and W) *Nutradiet*, low calorie	4 oz.	54
(S and W) *Nutradiet*, unsweetened	4 oz.	54
(Tillie Lewis)	½ cup	51
(White House)	½ cup	48
***APPLESAUCE CAKE MIX**, raisin (Duncan Hines)	1 cake	1800
APPLE TURNOVER (Pepperidge Farm)	3.3-oz. turnover	315
APRICOT:		
Whole	1 lb.	217
Canned, regular pack:		
(Del Monte)	½ cup	104
(Hunt's)	½ cup	103
(Stokely-Van Camp)	½ cup	103
Canned, low calorie:		
(Diet Delight)	½ cup	60
(S and W) *Nutradiet*, low calorie, whole	2 whole	31

*Prepared as Package Directs

Food and Description	Measure or Quantity	Calories
(S and W) *Nutradiet,* low calorie, halves	4 halves	40
(S and W) *Nutradiet,* unsweetened, halves	4 halves	38
(Tillie Lewis)	½ cup	49
Dehydrated, uncooked	4 oz.	376
Dried, uncooked (Del Monte)	½ cup	154

APRICOT-APPLE JUICE DRINK

(BC)	6 fl. oz.	96

APRICOT LIQUEUR (Leroux)

60 proof	1 fl. oz.	85

APRICOT NECTAR (Heinz)

	5½-fl.-oz. can	90

APRICOT PIE FILLING:

(Comstock)	1 cup	314
(Lucky Leaf)	8 oz.	316

APRICOT & PINEAPPLE NECTAR

(S and W) *Nutradiet*	4 oz.	35

APRICOT & PINEAPPLE PRESERVE:

Sweetened (Bama)	1 T.	54
Low calorie (Diet Delight)	1 T.	21

AQUAVIT (Leroux) 90 proof

	1 fl. oz.	75

ARTICHOKE, Globe or French:

Raw	1 lb.	85
Frozen, hearts (Birds Eye)	5-6 hearts	22

ASPARAGUS:

Raw	1 lb.	66
Canned:		
Cut spears & liq. (Green Giant)	10½-oz. can	48
Spears & liq. (Green Giant)	15-oz. can	69
Frozen:		
Cuts (Birds Eye)	10-oz. pkg.	60
Cut spears in butter sauce (Green Giant)	9-oz. pkg.	120

*Prepared as Package Directs

Food and Description	Measure or Quantity	Calories
Spears (Birds Eye)	10-oz. pkg.	66
Spears with Hollandaise sauce (Birds Eye)	10-oz. pkg.	291
AUNT JEMIMA SYRUP	8 fl. oz.	848
AVOCADO, whole	1 lb.	568
***AWAKE** (Birds Eye)	½ cup	55
AYDS	1 piece	26

B

Food and Description	Measure or Quantity	Calories
BAC ONION (Lawry's)	1 pkg.	372
*BAC*OS* (General Mills)	1 T.	29
BACON:		
Raw (Wilson)	8 oz.	1352
(Oscar Mayer) 11–14 slices per lb. raw	1 slice (cooked)	67
(Oscar Mayer) 18–26 slices per lb. raw	1 slice (cooked)	36
(Oscar Mayer) 25–30 slices per ¾ lb. raw	1 slice (cooked)	24
BACON BITS:		
(French's)	1 oz.	99
(McCormick)	1 oz.	113
BACON, CANADIAN:		
(Oscar Mayer)	1-oz. slice	45
(Wilson)	1-oz.	42
BAGEL, water or egg	3″ dia.	165
BAKING POWDER:		
(Calumet)	1 tsp.	2
(Royal)	1 tsp.	5
BAKON DELITES (Wise):		
Regular	½-oz. bag	72
Barbecue flavor	½-oz. bag	70

*Prepared as Package Directs

Food and Description	Measure or Quantity	Calories
BANANA:		
Common	1 lb.	262
Red	1 lb.	278
BANANA CAKE MIX:		
*(Betty Crocker) layer	1 cake	2870
*(Duncan Hines)	1 cake	2842
(Pillsbury)	1 oz.	120
(Pillsbury) loaf cake	1 oz.	117
BANANA EXTRACT, imitation:		
(Ehlers)	1 tsp.	7
(French's)	1 tsp.	20
BANANA PIE:		
Frozen (Mrs. Smith's)	8″ pie	1284
Frozen (Morton)	14.4-oz. pie	1026
BANANA PUDDING (Del Monte)	5-oz. can	187
BANANA PUDDING & PIE FILLING:		
*Instant (Jell-O)	½ cup	178
*Instant (Royal)	½ cup	176
*Regular (Jell-O)	½ cup	173
*Regular (My-T-Fine)	½ cup	175
*Regular (Royal)	½ cup	163
BARBECUE DINNER MIX:		
(Hunt's) *Skillet*	2-lb. 1-oz. pkg.	1404
*Without added fat (Lipton)	1 pkg.	720
BARDOLINO WINE (Antinori)		
12% alcohol	3 fl. oz.	84
BASS:		
Black sea, whole	1 lb.	165
Smallmouth & largemouth, whole	1 lb.	146
Striped, whole	1 lb.	205
White, whole	1 lb.	173
B and B LIQUEUR (Julius Wile)		
86 proof	1 fl. oz.	94

*Prepared as Package Directs

Food and Description	Measure or Quantity	Calories
BAVARIAN PIE FILLING		
(Lucky Leaf)	8 oz.	306
BAVARIAN PIE or PUDDING MIX:		
*Cream (My-T-Fine)	½ cup	175
*Custard *Rice-A-Roni*	4 oz.	143
BAVARIAN-STYLE BEANS &		
SPAETZLE (Birds Eye)	10-oz. pkg.	405
BEAN, BAKED:		
Canned with brown sugar sauce:		
(B & M) red kidney bean	1 cup	360
(B & M) yellow eye bean	1 cup	359
(Homemaker's) red kidney bean	1 cup	337
Canned in molasses sauce:		
(Heinz)	1 cup	283
& brown sugar sauce (Campbell)	1 cup	310
Canned with pork:		
(Campbell) Home Style	1 cup	302
(Hunt's) *Snack Pack*	5-oz. can	169
(Van Camp)	1 cup	286
Canned with pork & molasses sauce:		
(B & M) Michigan Pea, New		
England-style	1 cup	336
(Heinz) Boston-style	1 cup	303
(Homemaker's) Michigan Pea,		
New England-style	1 cup	320
Canned with pork & tomato sauce:		
(Campbell)	1 cup	262
(Heinz)	1 cup	293
(Libby's)	1 cup	286
Canned with tomato sauce:		
(Heinz) *Campside*	1 cup	350
(Heinz) vegetarian	1 cup	267
(Van Camp)	1 cup	276
BEAN & FRANKFURTER, canned:		
(Campbell) in tomato & molasses		
sauce	1 cup	364
(Heinz)	1 can	399
(Van Camp) *Beanie-Weenee*	1 cup	316

*Prepared as Package Directs

Food and Description	Measure or Quantity	Calories
BEAN & FRANKFURTER DINNER:		
(Banquet)	10¾-oz. dinner	687
(Morton)	12-oz. dinner	554
(Swanson)	11½-oz. dinner	610
BEAN, GREEN		
Whole	1 lb.	128
Canned, cut, solids & liq.		
(Comstock-Greenwood)	½ cup	20
Frozen:		
Cut (Birds Eye)	9-oz. pkg.	66
Whole (Birds Eye)	9-oz. pkg.	69
French-style (Birds Eye)	9-oz. pkg.	66
French-style with sliced		
mushrooms (Birds Eye)	9-oz. pkg.	78
French-style, with toasted		
almonds (Birds Eye)	9-oz. pkg.	156
In butter sauce (Green Giant)	9-oz. pkg.	96
In mushroom sauce (Green		
Giant)	10-oz. pkg.	126
BEAN, KIDNEY or RED:		
(Sinsheimer)	4 oz.	397
Canned, solids & liq.	½ cup	115
BEAN, LIMA, young:		
Raw, whole	1 lb.	223
Raw, without shell	1 lb.	558
Canned, solids & liq.		
(Stokely-Van Camp)	½ cup	82
Frozen:		
Baby butter beans (Birds Eye)	10-oz. pkg.	369
(Birds Eye)	10-oz. pkg.	333
In butter sauce (Green Giant)	10-oz. pkg.	324
Fordhooks (Birds Eye)	10-oz. pkg.	228
BEAN, LIMA, (Sinsheimer)	4 oz.	368
BEAN, PINTO (Sinsheimer)	4 oz.	397
BEAN, REFRIED, canned (Rosarita)	4 oz.	120

*Prepared as Package Directs

Food and Description	Measure or Quantity	Calories
BEAN SALAD:		
(Hunt's) *Snack Pack*	5-oz. can	111
(Le Sueur)	1-lb. 1-oz. can	276
BEAN, SEMI-MATURE, drained		
(B&M)	8¾-oz. can	310
BEAN SOUP, canned:		
*(Manischewitz)	1 can	222
*With smoked pork (Heinz)	1 cup	157
BEAN SOUP, BLACK:		
*(Campbell)	1 can	182
(Crosse & Blackwell)	1 can	192
BEAN SPROUT:		
Mung	½ lb.	80
Soy, raw	½ lb.	104
Canned (Mow Sang)	28-oz. can	79
BEAN, WHITE, NAVY or PEA		
(Sinsheimer)	4 oz.	396
BEAN, YELLOW or WAX:		
Raw	1 lb.	108
Canned:		
Golden, whole (Green Giant)	8.5-oz. can	26
Cut (Green Giant)	8.5-oz. can	38
Frozen, cut (Birds Eye)	9-oz. pkg.	72
BEAUJOLAIS WINE, French		
(B & G) 12% alcohol	3 fl. oz.	60
BEEF:		
Brisket:		
Raw, lean & fat	1 lb. (weighed with bone)	1284
Raw, lean & fat	1 lb. (weighed without bone)	1529
Chuck:		
Raw, lean & fat	1 lb. (weighed with bone)	984

*Prepared as Package Directs

Food and Description	Measure or Quantity	Calories
Raw, lean & fat	1 lb. (weighed without bone)	1166
Flank, raw, 100% lean	1 lb.	653
Foreshank, raw, lean & fat	1 lb. (weighed with bone)	531
Ground:		
Lean, raw	1 lb.	812
Regular, raw	1 lb.	1216
Heel of round, raw, lean & fat	1 lb.	966
Rib:		
Raw, lean & fat	1 lb. (weighed with bone)	1673
Raw, lean & fat	1 lb. (weighed without bone)	1819
Round:		
Raw, lean & fat	1 lb. (weighed with bone)	863
Raw, lean & fat	1 lb. (weighed without bone)	894
Rump:		
Raw, lean & fat	1 lb. (weighed with bone)	1167
Raw, lean & fat	1 lb. (weighed without bone)	1374
Steak, club:		
Raw, lean & fat	1 lb. (weighed with bone)	1443
Raw, lean & fat	1 lb. (weighed without bone)	1724
Steak, porterhouse, raw, lean & fat	1 lb. (weighed with bone)	1603
Steak, sirloin, double-bone:		
Raw, lean & fat	1 lb. (weighed with bone)	1240
Raw, lean & fat	1 lb. (weighed without bone)	1510
Steak, sirloin, hipbone:		
Raw, lean & fat	1 lb. (weighed with bone)	1585
Raw, lean & fat	1 lb. (weighed without bone)	1869

*Prepared as Package Directs

Steak, sirloin, wedge & round-bone:

Raw, lean & fat	1 lb. (weighed with bone)	1316
Raw, lean & fat	1 lb. (weighed without bone)	1420
Steak, T-bone, raw, lean & fat	1 lb. (weighed with bone)	1596
BEEFARONI (Chef Boy-Ar-Dee)	40-oz. can	1030

BEEF BOUILLON/BROTH:

(Croyden House) instant	1 tsp.	12
(Herb-Ox) (Steero)	1 cube	6
(Herb-Ox) instant	1 packet	8
*(Knorr Swiss)	6 fl. oz.	13
(Maggi) (Wyler's)	1 cube or 1 tsp.	7
(Wyler's) no salt added	1 cube	11

BEEF & CABBAGE, casserole (Mrs. Paul's)

	12-oz. pkg.	432

BEEF, CHIPPED:

(Armour Star)	1 oz.	48
Cooked (Oscar Mayer)	1 thin slice	7
Frozen, creamed (Banquet)	5-oz. bag	126

BEEF, CHOPPED or DICED, canned:

(Armour Star)	12-oz. can	1042
(Hormel)	12-oz. can	867

BEEF DINNER:

(Banquet)	11-oz. dinner	309
(Swanson)	11½-oz. dinner	371
(Swanson) 3-course	15-oz. dinner	567
Chopped (Banquet)	9-oz. dinner	386
Chopped sirloin (Swanson)	10-oz. dinner	447
Chopped (Weight Watchers)	18-oz. dinner	665
Sliced (Morton) 3-course	1-lb. 1-oz. dinner	563

BEEF & EGGPLANT (Mrs. Paul's)	12-oz. pkg.	420

*Prepared as Package Directs

Food and Description	Measure or Quantity	Calories
BEEF GOULASH:		
Canned (Heinz)	8½-oz. can	253
Seasoning mix (Lawry's)	1.7-oz. pkg.	127
BEEF & GREEN PEPPER, casserole		
(Mrs. Paul's)	12-oz. pkg.	386
BEEF, GROUND, seasoning mix:		
With onions (Durkee)	1⅛-oz. pkg.	92
With onions (French's)	1⅛-oz. pkg.	79
BEEF HASH, ROAST (Stouffer's)	11½-oz. pkg.	460
BEEF PATTIES, & BURGUNDY		
SAUCE, frozen (Morton House)	4¹⁄₆-oz. serving	153
BEEF PIE:		
(Banquet)	2-lb. 4-oz. pie	1311
(Stouffer's)	10-oz. pie	572
(Swanson)	16-oz. pie	703
BEEF PUFFS (Durkee)	1 piece	47
BEEF, SLICED, with barbecue sauce		
(Banquet)	5-oz. bag	152
BEEF SOUP:		
(Campbell)	1 can	370
Barley (Manischewitz)	1 can	166
Consommé (Campbell)	1 can	66
*Noodle (Heinz)	1 cup	74
Vegetable (Manischewitz)	1 can	118
BEEF SOUP MIX, noodle		
(Lipton) *Cup-a-Soup*	1 pkg.	34
BEEF STEW:		
(Armour Star)	24-oz. can	590
(Austex)	15½-oz. can	347
(Bunker Hill)	23-oz. can	634
(Heinz)	8½-oz. can	253
(Wilson)	15½-oz. can	343

*Prepared as Package Directs

Food and Description	Measure or Quantity	Calories
Dietetic (Claybourne)	8-oz. can	365
Dietetic (Slim-ette)	8-oz. can	195
Meatball (Hormel)	1-lb. 8-oz. can	631
Frozen:		
Buffet (Banquet)	2-lb. pkg.	720
Family (Tom Thumb)	3-lb. 8-oz. tray	1375

BEEF STEW SEASONING MIX:

(Durkee)	1 pkg. (1¾-oz.)	99
(French's)	1 pkg.	133
(Lawry's)	1 pkg.	131

BEEF STROGANOFF:

Canned (Hormel)	1-lb. can	645
Mix (Chef Boy-Ar-Dee)	6⅔-oz. pkg.	232
Mix (Hunt's) *Skillet*	1-lb. 2-oz. pkg.	794

BEER, regular:

Andeker	12 fl. oz.	165
Buckeye, 4.6% alcohol	12 fl. oz.	144
Budweiser, 4.9% alcohol	12 fl. oz.	156
Budweiser, 3.9% alcohol	12 fl. oz.	137
Busch Bavarian, 4.9% alcohol	12 fl. oz.	156
Busch Bavarian, 3.9% alcohol	12 fl. oz.	137
Eastside Lager	12 fl. oz.	145
Gold Medal	12 fl. oz.	160
Hamm's	12 fl. oz.	151
Knickerbocker, 4.6% alcohol	12 fl. oz.	160
Meister Brau Premium, 4.6% alcohol	12 fl. oz.	144
Meister Brau Premium Draft, 4.6% alcohol	12 fl. oz.	144
Michelob, 4.9% alcohol	12 fl. oz.	160
Narragansett, 4.7% alcohol	12 fl. oz.	155
North Star, regular	12 fl. oz.	165
North Star, 3.2 low gravity	12 fl. oz.	142
Pabst Blue Ribbon	12 fl. oz.	150
Pfeifer, regular	12 fl. oz.	165
Pfeifer, 3.2 low gravity	12 fl. oz.	142
Rheingold, 4.6% alcohol	12 fl. oz.	160
Schlitz	12 fl. oz.	155
Schmidt, regular, or extra special	12 fl. oz.	165

*Prepared as Package Directs

Food and Description	Measure or Quantity	Calories
Schmidt, 3.2 low gravity	12 fl. oz.	142
Utica Club	12 fl. oz.	150
Yuengling Premium	12 fl. oz.	144
BEER, low carbohydrate:		
Dia-beer	12 fl. oz.	145
Dia-beer	7 fl. oz.	85
Gablinger's, 4.5% alcohol	12 fl. oz.	99
Meister Brau Lite, 4.6% alcohol	12 fl. oz.	96
BEER, NEAR, *Kingsbury*		
(Heileman), 0.4% alcohol	12 fl. oz.	62
BEET:		
Without tops	1 lb.	137
Solids & liq., tiny, whole		
(Le Sueur)	1-lb. can	148
Solids & liq., slices (Libby's)	½ cup	34
Frozen, sliced, in orange flavor		
glaze (Birds Eye)	10-oz. pkg.	162
BENEDICTINE LIQUEUR (Julius		
Wile) 86 proof	1 fl. oz.	112
BIG WHEEL (Hostess)	1 cake	166
BISCUIT, egg (Stella D'oro):		
Dietetic or regular	1 piece	42
Roman	1 piece	135
Sugared	1 piece	59
BISCUIT DOUGH:		
*(Borden) Gem	1 biscuit	100
(Pillsbury) buttermilk,		
Tenderflake	1 oz.	94
(Pillsbury) *Hungry Jack*		
Butter Tastin'	1 oz.	101
BISCUIT MIX, *Bisquick*		
(Betty Crocker)	1 cup	503
BITTER LEMON:		
(Hoffman)	6 fl. oz.	85
(Schweppes)	6 fl. oz.	96

*Prepared as Package Directs

Food and Description	Measure or Quantity	Calories
BITTER ORANGE (Schweppes)	6 fl. oz.	92
BITTERS (Angostura)	1 tsp.	14
BLACKBERRY:		
Fresh, with hulls	1 lb.	250
Canned, heavy syrup	½ cup	118
Canned, low calorie		
(S and W) *Nutradiet*	4 oz.	41
BLACKBERRY PIE:		
(Tastykake)	4-oz. pie	386
Frozen (Banquet)	5-oz. serving	376
BLACKBERRY PIE FILLING,		
canned:		
(Comstock)	1 cup	438
(Lucky Leaf)	8 oz.	258
BLACK-EYED PEA, frozen		
(Birds Eye)	½ cup	92
BLOODY MARY MIX (Bar-Tender's)	1 serving	26
BLUEBERRY:		
Untrimmed	1 lb.	259
Quick thaw (Birds Eye)	½ cup	114
BLUEBERRY PIE:		
(Tastykake)	4-oz. pie	376
(Banquet)	5-oz. serving	366
(Morton)	20-oz. pie	1440
(Morton)	46-oz. pie	3088
(Mrs. Smith's)	8″ pie	1764
(Mrs. Smith's) natural juice	9″ pie	2912
(Mrs. Smith's)	10″ pie	3114
Tart (Pepperidge Farm)	3-oz. pie tart	277
BLUEBERRY PIE FILLING:		
(Comstock)	1 cup	332
(Lucky Leaf)	8 oz.	256
(Musselman's)	1 cup	321

*Prepared as Package Directs

Food and Description	Measure or Quantity	Calories
BLUEBERRY TURNOVER, frozen		
(Pepperidge Farm)	1 turnover	321
BLUEFISH, whole	1 lb.	271
BOLOGNA:		
All meat (Armour Star)	1-oz. slice	99
All meat (Eckrich)	1-oz. slice	92
All meat (Hormel)	1 oz.	85
All meat (Oscar Mayer)	1-oz. slice	89
Pure beef (Oscar Mayer)	.8-oz. slice	72
BORSCHT (Manischewitz)	1 cup	72
BOSCO (Best Foods)	1 T.	56
***BOSTON CREAM PIE MIX**		
(Betty Crocker)	1 pie	2120
BOYSENBERRY (S and W)		
Nutradiet	4 oz.	36
BOYSENBERRY PIE, frozen:		
(Banquet)	5-oz. serving	374
(Morton)	20-oz. pie	1494
BRAINS, all animals	1 lb.	568
BRAN BREAKFAST CEREAL:		
Plain:		
All-Bran (Kellogg's)	1 oz.	107
Bran Buds (Kellogg's)	1 oz.	106
40% bran flakes (Kellogg's)	1 oz.	109
40% bran flakes (Post)	1 oz.	97
100% bran (Nabisco)	1 oz.	97
Raisin bran flakes:		
(Kellogg's)	1 oz.	104
(Post)	1 oz.	92
Cinnamon (Post)	1 oz.	92
BRANDY, FLAVORED:		
Apricot (Bols) 70 proof	1 fl. oz.	100
Blackberry (Garnier) 70 proof	1 fl. oz.	86

*Prepared as Package Directs

Food and Description	Measure or Quantity	Calories
Cherry (Hiram Walker) 70 proof	1 fl. oz.	86
Coffee (Leroux) coffee & brandy,		
70 proof	1 fl. oz.	91
Ginger (Old Mr. Boston) 70 proof	1 fl. oz.	74
Peach (Mr. Boston's)		
peach & brandy, 42 proof	1 fl. oz.	75
BRATWURST (Oscar Mayer)	1-oz. slice	94
BRAUNSCHWEIGER:		
(Oscar Mayer)	1-oz. slice	107
(Wilson)	1-oz. slice	90
Beef (Eckrich)	1-oz. slice	71
Liver cheese (Oscar Mayer)	3-oz. slice	102
BRAZIL NUT, Whole	4 oz.	356
BREAD:		
Cheese, party (Pepperidge Farm)	6-gram slice	18
Cracked-wheat (Pepperidge Farm)	.9-oz. slice	69
Daffodil Farm (Wonder)	.8-oz. slice	58
Date-nut loaf (Thomas')	1.1-oz. slice	94
Finn Crisp	1 piece	22
French (Pepperidge Farm)	1″ slice	87
Glutogen Gluten (Thomas')	.5-oz. slice	35
Italian (Pepperidge Farm)	1″ slice	90
King's Bread (Wasa)	3.5-oz. slice	365
Natural Health (Arnold)	.9-oz. slice	73
Oatmeal:		
(Arnold)	.8-oz. slice	64
(Pepperidge Farm)	.9-oz. slice	68
Panettone (Van de Kamp's)	1½-lb. loaf	2167
Profile, dark (Wonder)	.8 oz. slice	55
Profile, light (Wonder)	.8-oz. slice	57
Protogen Protein (Thomas')	.7-oz. slice	46
Pumpernickel:		
(Arnold) Jewish	1.4-oz. slice	104
(Levy's)	1.1-oz. slice	70
(Pepperidge Farm) family	1.2-oz. slice	79
(Pepperidge Farm) party	8-gram slice	20
(Wonder)	.8-oz. slice	54
Raisin:		
Cinnamon (Pepperidge Farm)	.9-oz. slice	74

*Prepared as Package Directs

Food and Description	Measure or Quantity	Calories
Cinnamon (Thomas') (Wonder)	.8-oz. slice	60
Rite Diet (Thomas')	.7-oz. slice	50
Roman Meal	.8-oz. slice	63
Rye:		
(Arnold) Melba thin, Jewish	.6-oz. slice	43
(Arnold) Jewish, seeded or unseeded	1.2-oz. slice	94
(Levy's) with or without caraway	1.1-oz. slice	70
(Levy's) Westchester, with or without seeds	1.1-oz. slice	55
(Pepperidge Farm) family	1.2-oz. slice	82
(Pepperidge Farm) party	6-gram slice	16
(Pepperidge Farm) seedless	1.2-oz. slice	82
Ry-King (Wasa):		
Brown	1 piece	43
Golden	1 piece	33
Lite	1 piece	30
Seasoned	1 piece	39
(Wonder)	.8-oz. slice	55
Soy & wheat:		
(Mannafood)	.9-oz. slice	65
Salt free (Mannafood)	.9-oz. slice	60
Sprouted wheat (Mannafood)	1-oz. slice	58
Wheat germ (Pepperidge Farm)	.9-oz. slice	68
White		
(Arnold) Melba thin	.5-oz. slice	43
(Arnold) sandwich	.9-oz. slice	70
(Pepperidge Farm):		
Large loaf, Calif. only	.8-oz. slice	66
Very thin slice, East	.5-oz. slice	42
Very thin slice, Mid-west	.6-oz. slice	42
Brick Oven (Arnold) 1-lb. loaf	.8-oz. slice	68
Hearthstone (Arnold) 1-lb. loaf	.9-oz. slice	71
Whole-wheat *Brick Oven* 1-lb. loaf	.8-oz. slice	65
BREAD, CANNED:		
Banana nut (Dromedary)	½" slice	75
Brown, plain (B & M)	½" slice	83
Brown with raisins (B & M)	½" slice	78
Chocolate nut (Dromedary)	½" slice	86

*Prepared as Package Directs

Food and Description	Measure or Quantity	Calories
Date & nut (Crosse & Blackwell)	½" slice	65
Date & nut (Dromedary)	½" slice	74
Orange nut (Dromedary)	½" slice	78

BREAD CRUMBS:

(Old London)	1 cup	468
Seasoned (Contadina)	1 cup	397

BREAD STICK:

Cheese or salt (Keebler)	1 piece	10
Dietetic (Stella D'oro)	1 piece	39
Garlic or sesame (Keebler)	1 piece	11
Onion (Stella D'oro)	1 piece	42
Regular (Stella D'oro)	1 piece	40

BREAD STUFFING MIX:

Corn bread (Pepperidge Farm)	8-oz. pkg.	836
Cube (Pepperidge Farm)	7-oz. pkg.	756
Herb seasoned (Pepperidge Farm)	8-oz. bag	836

BROADBEAN, Italian bean (Birds
Eye) 9-oz. pkg. 69

BROCCOLI:

Raw	1 lb.	113
Cut (Birds Eye)	10-oz. pkg.	81
Spears (Birds Eye)	10-oz. pkg.	78
In butter sauce (Green Giant)	10-oz. pkg.	153
In cheese sauce (Green Giant)	10-oz. pkg.	189
In Hollandaise sauce (Birds Eye)	10-oz. pkg.	300

BROTWURST (Oscar Mayer) 3-oz. link 275

BRUSSELS SPROUT:

Raw	1 lb.	188
Au gratin, casserole (Green Giant)	10-oz. pkg.	210
Baby sprouts (Birds Eye)	10-oz. pkg.	102
In butter sauce (Green Giant)	10-oz. pkg.	165

BUCKWHEAT GROATS:

(Pocono)	1 oz.	104
Wolff's Kasha (Birkett)	1 oz.	108

*Prepared as Package Directs

Food and Description	Measure or Quantity	Calories
BUC WHEATS (General Mills)	1 cup	102
BULGUR, canned	8 oz.	382
BURGUNDY WINE:		
(Italian Swiss Colony-Gold Medal)		
12.3% alcohol	3 fl. oz.	63
(Taylor) 12½% alcohol	3 fl. oz.	72
BURGUNDY WINE, SPARKLING:		
(B & G) 12% alcohol	3 fl. oz.	69
(Chanson)	3 fl. oz.	72
(Gold Seal) 12% alcohol	3 fl. oz.	87
BURRITOS (Rosarita)	8-oz. pkg.	486
BUTTER:		
Regular	1 stick	812
Whipped	1 stick	544
***BUTTER BRICKLE LAYER CAKE**		
MIX (Betty Crocker)	1 cake	2436
BUTTERFISH:		
Gulf, Whole	1 lb.	220
Northern, Whole	1 lb.	391
BUTTERSCOTCH MORSELS		
(Nestlé's)	6-oz. pkg.	900
BUTTERSCOTCH PIE (Banquet)	2½-oz. serving	187
BUTTERSCOTCH PUDDING:		
Chilled (Breakstone)	5-oz. container	252
Chilled (Sealtest)	4 oz.	124
(Del Monte)	5-oz. can	191
(Hunt's)	5-oz. can	238
(Sanna) *Swiss Miss*	5-oz. container	145
BUTTERSCOTCH PUDDING or		
PIE MIX:		
Sweetened:		
*Instant (Jell-O)	½ cup	178
*Instant (Royal)	½ cup	176

*Prepared as Package Directs

*Regular (Jell-O)	½ cup	173
*Regular (My-T-Fine)	½ cup	175
*Regular (Royal)	½ cup	191
*Low calorie (D-Zerta)	½ cup	107

C

CABBAGE:

White	1 lb.	86
Red	1 lb.	111
Savoy	1 lb.	86
CABBAGE, CHINESE or CELERY	1 lb.	62
CABBAGE ROLLS, stuffed (Holloway House)	7 oz. roll	184
CABBAGE, SPOON or WHITE MUSTARD or PAKCHOY	1 lb.	69
CAKE DECORATOR (Pillsbury)	1 oz.	110

CAKE ICING (Betty Crocker):

Butterscotch	16.5-oz. can	1968
Chocolate	16.5-oz. can	1944
Dark Dutch fudge	16.5-oz. can	1836
Lemon or vanilla	16.5-oz. can	1992

CAKE ICING MIX (Betty Crocker):

Cherry, creamy	1 cake's icing	1668
Coconut-pecan	1 cake's icing	1224
Coconut, toasted	1 cake's icing	1692
Orange	1 cake's icing	1608
Spice	1 cake's icing	1668
White, fluffy	1 cake's icing	696

CAKE MIX:

White:

*(Betty Crocker)	1 cake	2280
*(Duncan Hines)	1 cake	2280
(Pillsbury)	1 oz.	121
*(Swans Down)	1 cake	2124

*Prepared as Package Directs

Food and Description	Measure or Quantity	Calories
Yellow:		
*(Betty Crocker)	1 cake	2424
*Golden butter (Duncan Hines)	1 cake	3396
*(Swans Down)	1 cake	2232

CANDY:

Almonds, candy-coated (Hershey's)	1 oz.	142
Almond cluster (Peter Paul)	1³/₁₆-oz. pkg.	171
Almond Joy (Peter Paul)	1¾-oz. pkg.	231
Baby Ruth (Curtiss)	1 oz.	135
Baffle Bar (Cardinet's)	1¾-oz. bar	189
Black Crows (Mason)	1 oz.	100
Bridge mix (Nabisco)	1 piece	8
Butterfinger (Curtiss)	1 oz.	134
Candy corn (Brach's)	1 piece	7
Caramel, chocolate or vanilla (Kraft)	1 piece	33
Caravelle (Peter Pan)	1½-oz. pkg.	190
Cashew crunch, canned (Planters)	1 oz.	134
Charleston Chew	10¢ size	149
Cherry, chocolate-covered		
(Brach's) (Nabisco)	1 piece	66
Chocolate bar:		
Milk chocolate:		
(Ghirardelli)	1.1-oz. bar	169
(Hershey's)	1 oz.	156
Semisweet (Nestlé's)	1 oz.	141
Chocolate bar with almonds:		
(Ghirardelli)	1.1-oz. bar·	173
(Nestlé's)	1 oz.	149
Chocolate block, milk (Hershey's)	1 oz.	145
Chuckles	1 oz.	92
Cluster, peanut (Brach's)	1 piece	79
Coconut:		
Bon Bons (Brach's)	1 piece	70
Cream Egg (Hershey's)	1 oz.	142
Fiddle Faddle	1½-oz. packet	177
5th Avenue Bar (Luden's)	15¢ size	179
Fudge:		
(Nabisco) *Home Style*	1 piece	90
(Tom Houston)	1.5-oz. bar	179
Good & Plenty	1 oz.	100

*Prepared as Package Directs

Food and Description	Measure or Quantity	Calories
Hard candy:		
(Reed's)	1 piece	17
Sour balls (Brach's)	1 piece	22
Hollywood	1½-oz. bar	183
Jelly beans (Heide)	1 oz.	90
Jujyfruits (Heide)	1 oz.	94
Kisses (Hershey's)	1 piece	25
Krackel Bar (Hershey's)	1 oz.	152
Licorice twist (American		
Licorice Co):		
Black	1 piece	27
Red	1 piece	33
Life Saver (Beech-Nut)	1 drop	10
Malted Milk Balls (Brach's)	1 piece	9
Mars Almond Bar (M & M/Mars)	1 oz.	130
Marshmallow (Campfire)	1 oz.	111
Mary Jane (Miller)	5¢ size	125
Milky Way	1 oz.	120
Mint or peppermint:		
Afterdinner (Richardson)	1 oz.	109
Mason Mints	1 oz.	200
(Nabisco)	½-oz. piece	64
Mounds (Peter Paul)	1⁹/₁₀-oz. pkg.	236
M & M's (M & M/Mars) plain or		
peanut	1 oz.	140
Mr. Goodbar (Hershey's)	1 oz.	157
Necco Wafers	1 piece	7
$100,000 Bar (Nestlé's)	1 oz.	121
Orange slices (Nabisco) *Chuckles*	1 piece	29
Peanut, chocolate-covered		
(Brach's)	1 piece	11
Peanut Block Bar (Planter's)	1 oz.	139
Peanut butter cup (Reese's)	1 oz.	143
Raisin, chocolate-covered (BB)	5¢-size pkg.	140
Spearmint leaves (Quaker City)	1 oz.	107
Sugar Daddy (Nabisco):		
Caramel	1-lb. pkg.	1809
Choco-flavored	.4-oz. piece	51
Nugget	.4-oz. piece	48
Taffy, salt water (Brach's)	1 piece	31
Tootsie Roll	1¢ size or midgee	26
Variety pack (Nabisco) *Chuckles*	2-oz. pack	206

*Prepared as Package Directs

Food and Description	Measure or Quantity	Calories

CANDY, DIETETIC:
Almonds, chocolate-covered (Estee)	1 piece	22
Chocolate, assorted, *Slimtreats*	1 piece	13
Chocolate bar with almonds (Estee)	¾-oz. bar	127
Chocolate bar, milk (Estee)	¾-oz. bar	126
Gum drops, assorted (Estee)	1 piece	3
Hard candy, assorted (Estee)	1 piece	12
Mint (Estee)	1 piece	4
Petit fours (Estee)	1 piece	48
TV mix (Estee)	1 piece	11

CANTALOUPE, whole — 1 lb. — 68

CAPERS (Crosse & Blackwell) — 1 T. — 6

CAP'N CRUNCH:
(Quaker)	1 oz.	123
Crunchberries (Quaker)	1 oz.	119
Peanut butter (Quaker)	1 oz.	128

*CARAMEL CAKE MIX (Duncan Hines) — 1 cake — 2424

CARAMEL PUDDING (My-T-Fine) — 5-oz. can — 184

CARAWAY SEED — 1 oz. — 72

CARNATION INSTANT BREAKFAST:
Chocolate, coffee or vanilla	1 pkg.	128
Special Morning, strawberry	1 pkg.	188

CARP, whole, raw — 1 lb. — 156

CARROT:
Raw	1 lb.	156
Canned (Stokely-Van Camp)	½ cup	32
Frozen:		
Honey glazed (Green Giant)	10-oz. pkg.	213
In butter sauce (Green Giant)	10-oz. pkg.	150
With brown sugar glaze (Birds Eye)	10-oz. pkg.	261

*Prepared as Package Directs

Food and Description	Measure or Quantity	Calories
CASABA MELON	1 lb.	61
CASHEW NUT:		
Dry roasted (Flavor House)	1 oz.	172
Oil roasted (Skippy)	1 oz.	177
CATFISH, raw, fillet	1 lb.	468
CATSUP, regular:		
(Bama)	½ pt.	304
(Del Monte)	½ pt.	320
(Heinz)	½ pt.	256
(Hunt's)	½ pt.	288
(Stokely-Van Camp)	½ pt.	304
CATSUP, dietetic pack (Tillie Lewis)	½ pt.	112
CAULIFLOWER:		
Raw, flowerbuds	1 lb.	122
(Birds Eye)	10-oz. pkg.	63
Au gratin (Stouffer's)	10-oz. pkg.	339
In butter sauce (Green Giant)	10-oz. pkg.	111
CAULIFLOWER, PICKLED		
(Smucker's)	1 bud	24
CAVIAR, STURGEON:		
Pressed	1 oz.	90
Whole	1 oz.	74
CELERY, fresh, whole	1 lb.	58
CERTS (Warner-Lambert)	1 piece	6
CERVELAT:		
Dry	1 oz.	128
Soft	1 oz.	87
CHABLIS WINE:		
(B & G) 12% alcohol	3 fl. oz.	60
(Chanson) 11½% alcohol	3 fl. oz.	81
(Great Western)	3 fl. oz.	69

*Prepared as Package Directs

Food and Description	Measure or Quantity	Calories
CHAMPAGNE:		
(Bollinger)	3 fl. oz.	72
(Great Western) brut, 12.5% alcohol	3 fl. oz.	75
(Great Western) extra dry, 12.5% alcohol	3 fl. oz.	78
(Lejon) pink, 12% alcohol	3 fl. oz.	69
(Mogen David) 12% alcohol	3 fl. oz.	90
(Mumm's) extra dry, 12% alcohol	3 fl. oz.	82
(Veuve Clicquot) 12½% alcohol	3 fl. oz.	78
CHARD, Swiss, raw, whole	1 lb.	104
CHEERIOS (General Mills)	1 oz.	112
CHEESE:		
American or cheddar, natural:		
(Foremost Blue Moon)	1-oz. slice	100
(Kraft)	1 oz.	113
Cheddar (Sealtest)	1 oz.	115
Grated (Kraft)	1 oz.	129
Shredded (Kraft)	1 oz.	113
Sharp cheddar, *Wispride*	1 T.	50
American or cheddar, process:		
(Borden)	¾-oz. slice	83
(Kraft) (Sealtest)	1 oz.	105
Bleu or Blue:		
(Frigo) (Kraft)	1 oz.	99
Wispride	1 oz.	98
Blufort (Borden)	1¼-oz. pkg.	131
Brick (Kraft) process	1 oz.	101
Camembert (Borden) (Kraft)	1 oz.	86
Caraway (Kraft)	1 oz.	111
Colby (Borden) (Kraft)	1 oz.	111
Cottage, creamed, unflavored:		
(Borden)	8-oz. container	240
(Kraft)	8-oz. container	216
California (Breakstone)	8-oz. container	216
Light n' Lively (Sealtest)	1 cup	155
Low fat (Breakstone)	8-oz. container	184
Tangy or tiny curd (Breakstone)	8-oz. container	216
Cottage, creamed, flavored:		
Chive (Sealtest)	1 cup	211

*Prepared as Package Directs

Food and Description	Measure or Quantity	Calories
Pineapple (Sealtest)	1 cup	222
Spring Garden Salad (Sealtest)	1 cup	208
Cottage, uncreamed:		
Pot (Borden)	8-oz. pkg.	195
Skim milk (Breakstone)	8-oz. container	182
Cream cheese:		
Plain (Kraft):		
Philadelphia	1 oz.	104
Philadelphia, imitation	1 oz.	52
Flavored, chive (Borden)	1 oz.	96
Flavored, whipped (Kraft):		
Bacon & horseradish	1 oz.	96
Smoked salmon	1 oz.	90
Edam (House of Gold) (Kraft)	1 oz.	105
Gjetost (Kraft)	1 oz.	134
Gouda, baby (Foremost Blue Moon)	1 oz.	120
Gruyère (Borden) *Swiss Knight*	1 oz.	101
Liederkranz (Borden)	1 oz.	86
Monterey Jack (Borden) (Frigo)		
(Kraft)	1 oz.	103
Mozzarella:		
(Borden)	1 oz.	96
Skim, pizza (Kraft)	1 oz.	79
Muenster (Borden)	1 oz.	85
Old English (Kraft)	1 oz.	105
Parmesan, grated (Buitoni)	1 oz.	118
Parmesan & Romano, grated		
(Borden)	1 oz.	135
Pimento American (Kraft)	1 oz.	103
Pizza (Frigo)	1 oz.	73
Port du Salut (Foremost Blue		
Moon)	1 oz.	100
Provolone (Frigo) (Kraft)	1 oz.	99
Ricotta (Sierra)	1 oz.	50
Roquefort (Borden)	1 oz.	107
Swiss, domestic:		
Natural (Borden) (Foremost Blue		
Moon) (Kraft) (Sealtest)	1 oz.	104
Process:		
(Borden)	1-oz. slice	96
(Borden)	¾-oz. slice	74
Swiss, imported, natural:		
(Borden)	1 oz.	104

*Prepared as Package Directs

Food and Description	Measure or Quantity	Calories
CHEESE CAKE (Mrs. Smith's)	8″ cake	1281
*CHEESE CAKE MIX:		
(Jell-O)	1 cake including crust	2040
(Royal) *No-Bake*	9″ cake including crust	2224
CHEESE FOOD:		
American, slices (Kraft)	1 oz.	94
Links (Kraft) *Handi-Snack,* bacon, garlic, jalapeño, *Nippy, Smokelle*	1 oz.	93
Loaf, *Pizzalone* (Kraft)	1 oz.	90
Pimento, slices (Kraft)	1 oz.	94
Swiss (Borden) (Kraft)	1 oz.	92
CHEESE PIE, pineapple (Mrs. Smith's)	8″ pie	1638
CHEESE PUFF (Durkee)	1 piece	59
CHEESE SOUFFLE (Stouffer's)	12-oz. pkg.	729
CHEESE SPREAD:		
(Borden) *Vera Sharp*	1 oz.	72
Bacon (Kraft) *Squeez-A-Snak*	1 oz.	83
Blue (Borden) *Vera Blue*	1 oz.	91
Cheez Whiz (Kraft)	1 oz.	76
Neufchâtel, clam (Kraft) *Party Snacks*	1 oz.	67
Onion, French (Nabisco) *Snack Mate*	1 tsp.	15
Velveeta (Kraft)	1 oz.	84
CHEESE STRAW, frozen (Durkee)	1 piece	29
CHERRY:		
Sour:		
Fresh	1 lb.	213
Canned, water pack, (Stokely-Van Camp)	½ cup	49
Sweet:		
Fresh	1 lb.	286

*Prepared as Package Directs

Canned, heavy syrup:		
With pits, Royal Anne		
(Del Monte)	½ cup	109
Pitted (Del Monte)	½ cup	92
Canned, dietetic pack, pitted:		
(Blue Boy)	4 oz.	52
(Tillie Lewis)	½ cup	65
Frozen (Birds Eye)	½ cup	122

*CHERRY CAKE (Duncan Hines)   1 cake   2316

CHERRY, CANDIED (Liberty)   1 oz.   93

CHERRY HEERING (Hiram Walker)
49 proof   1 fl. oz.   80

CHERRY, MARASCHINO (Liberty)   1 average cherry   8

CHERRY PIE:

(Hostess)	4½-oz. pie	337
Frozen:		
(Morton)	20-oz. pie	1500
(Mrs. Smith's)	8" pie	1852
Tart (Pepperidge Farm)	3-oz. pie tart	277

CHERRY PIE FILLING:

(Comstock)	1 cup	334
(Lucky Leaf)	8 oz.	242

CHERRY SOFT DRINK:

Sweetened:		
(Canada Dry)	6 fl. oz.	96
(Clicquot Club) (Cott) (Mission)	6 fl. oz.	94
(Dr. Brown's) (Key Food)		
(Nedick's) (Waldbaum)	6 fl. oz.	81
(Fanta)	6 fl. oz.	85
(Hoffman)	6 fl. oz.	87
(Shasta)	6 fl. oz.	88
(White Rock)	6 fl. oz.	89
(Yoo-Hoo)	6 fl. oz.	90
High-protein (Yoo-Hoo)	6 fl. oz.	114
(Yukon Club)	6 fl. oz.	86

*Prepared as Package Directs

Food and Description	Measure or Quantity	Calories
Unsweetened or low calorie:		
(Clicquot Club) (Cott)		
(Dr. Brown's) (Hoffman)		
(Key Food) (Mission)		
(No-Cal) (Waldbaum)		
(Yukon Club)	6 fl. oz.	2
(Shasta)	6 fl. oz.	<1
CHERRY TURNOVER (Pepperidge Farm)	3.3-oz. turnover	342
CHESTNUT, in shell	4 oz.	178
CHEWING GUM:		
Bazooka, bubble	5¢ size	85
Beech-Nut	1 stick	10
Chiclets	5¢ pkg.	65
Spearmint (Wrigley's)	1 stick	8
CHIANTI WINE:		
(Antinori) 12½% alcohol	3 fl. oz.	87
(Italian Swiss-Colony Gold Medal) 12.1% alcohol	3 fl. oz.	65
CHICKEN, raw, with bones:		
Capon, ready-to-cook	1 lb.	937
Fryer:		
Ready-to-cook	1 lb.	382
Back	1 lb.	385
Breast	1 lb.	394
Leg or drumstick	1 lb.	313
Neck	1 lb.	329
Rib	1 lb.	287
Thigh	1 lb.	435
Wing	1 lb.	325
Hen & cock, ready-to-cook	1 lb.	987
Roaster, ready-to-cook	1 lb.	791
CHICKEN A LA KING:		
Canned (Richardson & Robbins)	1 cup	272
Frozen (Banquet)	5-oz. bag	140
CHICKEN CACCIATORE (Hormel)	1-lb can	386

*Prepared as Package Directs

Food and Description	Measure or Quantity	Calories
CHICKEN, CANNED:		
(Lynden Farms) with broth	11-oz. jar	490
(Swanson) with broth	5-oz. can	223
CHICKEN, CREAMED (Stouffer's)	11½-oz. can	613
CHICKEN DINNER:		
Noodle (Heinz)	8½-oz. can	186
Noodle (Lynden Farms)	14-oz. jar	413
(Weight Watchers)	10-oz. luncheon	284
Boneless chicken (Swanson)		
Hungry Man	19-oz. dinner	746
Chicken & dumplings:		
Buffet (Banquet)	2-lb. pkg.	1306
(Morton)	12-oz. dinner	372
(Morton) 3-course	1-lb 5-oz. dinner	768
(Tom Thumb)	3-lb. 8-oz. tray	1920
Creole (Weight Watchers)	12-oz. luncheon	211
Fried:		
(Banquet)	11-oz. dinner	542
(Morton)	11-oz. dinner	482
(Morton) 3-course	1-lb. 1-oz. dinner	868
(Swanson)	11½-oz. dinner	600
(Swanson) 3-course	15-oz. dinner	639
With shoestring potato (Swanson)	25-oz. pkg.	1879
CHICKEN DIP (Durkee)	1 pkg.	286
CHICKEN FRICASSEE:		
Canned (College Inn)	1 cup	234
Canned (Richardson & Robbins)	1 cup	256
CHICKEN, FRIED (Banquet)	2-lb. chicken	2195
CHICKEN LIVER, chopped (Mrs. Kornberg's)	6-oz. pkg.	260
CHICKEN LIVER puff (Durkee)	1 piece	48
CHICKEN & NOODLES:		
(Banquet) buffet	2-lb. pkg.	735
Escalloped (Stouffer's)	11½-oz. pkg.	589

*Prepared as Package Directs

Food and Description	Measure or Quantity	Calories
CHICKEN PIE:		
(Banquet)	2-lb. 4-oz. pie	1408
(Stouffer's)	10-oz. pkg.	722
(Swanson) deep dish	16-oz. pie	708
CHICKEN PUFF (Durkee)	1 piece	49
CHICKEN SOUP:		
Broth:		
(Campbell)	1 can	106
(College Inn)	1 cup	30
*Dietetic (Claybourne)	8 oz.	9
Cream of (Heinz) *Great American*	1 cup	108
*Noodle (Manischewitz)	1 can	92
Rice (Campbell)	1 can	98
*Vegetable (Heinz)	1 cup	85
CHICKEN SOUP MIX:		
Noodle (Lipton) *Cup-a-Soup*	1 pkg.	38
With chicken (Lipton) *Cup-a-Soup*	1-oz. pkg.	42
CHICKEN SPREAD:		
(Swanson)	5-oz. can	283
(Underwood)	4¾-oz. can	301
CHICK PEA or GARBANZO, dry	1 lb.	1633
CHICORY, WITLOOF, Belgian or French endive	1 lb.	60
CHILI or CHILI CON CARNE:		
Canned, with beans:		
(Armour Star)	15½-oz. can	692
(Austex)	15½-oz. can	584
(Wilson)	15½-oz. can	630
Canned without beans:		
(Armour Star)	15½-oz. can	835
(Austex)	15½-oz. can	851
(Wilson)	15½-oz. can	840
***CHILI DOG SAUCE MIX**		
(McCormick)	.9-oz. serving	18

*Prepared as Package Directs

Food and Description	Measure or Quantity	Calories
CHILI SAUCE:		
(Del Monte)	½ pt.	288
(Heinz)	½ pt.	272
(Hunt's)	½ pt.	304
(Stokely-Van Camp)	½ pt.	240
CHILI SEASONING MIX:		
Chili-O (French's)	1¾-oz. pkg.	123
(Lawry's)	1.6-oz. pkg.	137
CHINESE DINNER, Egg Foo Young		
or Shrimp Chow Mein (Chun King)	11-oz. dinner	340
CHITTERLINGS (Hormel)	1-lb. 2-oz. can	832
CHOCOLATE, BAKING:		
Bitter:		
(Baker's)	1-oz. sq.	136
Pre-melted, *Choco-Bake*	1-oz. packet	172
(Hershey's)	1 oz.	183
Sweetened:		
Chips, milk (Hershey's)	1 oz.	156
Chips, semisweet (Baker's)	¼ cup	191
Chips, semisweet (Ghirardelli)	⅓ cup	299
Chips, semisweet (Hershey's)	1 oz.	152
German's, sweet (Baker's)	1 oz.	141
Morsels, milk (Nestlé's)	1 oz.	152
Morsels, semisweet (Nestlé's)	6-oz. pkg.	820
Morsels, semisweet (Nestlé's)	1 oz.	137
Semisweet (Baker's)	1-oz. sq.	132
CHOCOLATE CAKE:		
(Sara Lee)	1 oz.	102
Fudge (Pepperidge Farm)	18-oz. cake	1890
German (Sara Lee)	1 oz.	91
Golden (Pepperidge Farm)	18-oz. cake	1920
Pecan (Van de Kamp's)	2 layer	3366
CHOCOLATE CAKE MIX:		
*Chocolate malt layer (Betty Crocker)	1 cake	2400
*Deep chocolate (Duncan Hines)	1 cake	2412
*German chocolate (Swans Down)	1 cake	2244

*Prepared as Package Directs

Food and Description	Measure or Quantity	Calories
CHOCOLATE DRINK (Borden)	9½-fl.-oz. can	232
CHOCOLATE DRINK MIX, *Quik* (Nestlé's)	2 heaping tsps.	56
CHOCOLATE ICE CREAM:		
(Borden) 9.5% fat	¼ pt.	126
(Meadow Gold) 10% fat	¼ pt.	128
(Prestige) French	¼ pt.	182
(Sealtest)	¼ pt.	136
CHOCOLATE PIE:		
(Mrs. Smith's)	8″ pie	1484
Tart (Pepperidge Farm)	3-oz. pie tart	306
Velvet nut (Kraft)	16¾-oz. pie	1818
CHOCOLATE PUDDING:		
Chilled (Breakstone)	5-oz. container	256
Canned (Hunt's)	5-oz. can	239
CHOCOLATE PUDDING or PIE FILLING MIX:		
Regular:		
*(My-T-Fine)	½ cup	187
*(Royal)	½ cup	196
*Instant (Jell-O)	½ cup	190
*Low calorie (D-Zerta)	½ cup	102
CHOCOLATE RENNET MIX:		
(Junket)	1 tablet	1
CHOCOLATE SOFT DRINK		
Sweetened:		
(Clicquot Club) (Cott) (Mission)	6 fl. oz.	92
(Hoffman) *Cocoa Cooler*	6 fl. oz.	89
(Hoffman) (Yukon Club)	6 fl. oz.	87
(Yoo Hoo)	6 fl. oz.	90
(Yoo Hoo) High protein	6 fl. oz.	114
Low calorie:		
(Cliquot Club) (Cott) (Mission)	6 fl. oz.	2
(Hoffman) (Shasta)	6 fl. oz.	1
(No-Cal)	6 fl. oz.	3

*Prepared as Package Directs

Food and Description	Measure or Quantity	Calories
CHOCO-NUT SUNDAE CONE		
(Sealtest)	2½ fl. oz.	186
CHOP SUEY:		
Canned:		
Chicken (Mow Sang)	20-oz. can	113
Pork (Mow Sang)	20-oz. can	167
Frozen, beef (Banquet)	2-lb. pkg.	554
CHOW CHOW (Crosse &		
Blackwell)	1 T.	6
CHOW MEIN:		
Beef (Chun King) *Divider-Pak*	28-oz. can	440
Chicken (Chun King) *Divider-Pak*	28-oz. can	400
Pork (Chun King) *Divider-Pak*	28-oz. can	640
Frozen, chicken:		
(Banquet)	2-lb. pkg.	563
(Chun King)	15 oz.	280
CHUTNEY, *Major Grey's*	1 T.	53
CITRON, CANDIED (Liberty)	1 oz.	93
CLACKERS (General Mills)	1 oz.	111
CLAM:		
Raw, hard or round	1 lb.	71
Raw, soft	1 lb.	142
Chopped & minced, solids &		
liq. (Doxsee)	8 oz.	118
Steamed (Doxsee)	1-pt. 8 fl.-oz. can	152
Frozen, fried (Mrs. Paul's)	4 oz.	404
CLAM CHOWDER:		
Manhattan:		
(Crosse & Blackwell)	13-oz. can	122
(Snow)	8 oz.	85
New England:		
(Crosse & Blackwell)	13-oz. can	202
(Snow)	8 oz.	148
CLAM COCKTAIL (Sau-Sea)	4-oz. jar	80

*Prepared as Package Directs

Food and Description	Measure or Quantity	Calories
CLAM JUICE (Snow)	8 oz.	31
CLARET WINE (Gold Seal)		
12% alcohol	3 fl. oz.	82
CLORETS	1 piece	6
CLUB SODA SOFT DRINK, regular or dietetic, any brand	6 fl. oz.	0
COCOA, dry:		
(Droste)	1 T.	21
(Hershey's)	1-oz. packet	122
COCOA KRISPIES (Kellogg's)	1 oz.	111
COCOA MIX:		
(Nestlé's) *EverReady*	3 heaping tsp.	105
Instant, rich chocolate (Carnation)	1-oz. pkg.	109
COCOA PEBBLES (Post)	1 oz.	111
COCOA PUFFS (General Mills)	1 oz.	109
COCONUT:		
Fresh, whole	1 lb.	816
Dried:		
Angel Flake (Baker's)	½ cup	178
Cookie (Baker's)	½ cup	280
Crunchies (Baker's)	½ cup	352
Premium shred (Baker's)	½ cup	210
Southern-style (Baker's)	½ cup	170
COCONUT CAKE (Pepperidge Farm)	18-oz. cake	1938
***COCONUT CAKE MIX** (Duncan Hines)	1 cake	2400
COCONUT PIE:		
Cream:		
(Morton)	14.4-oz. pie	1112
(Mrs. Smith's)	8" pie	1400

*Prepared as Package Directs

Food and Description	Measure or Quantity	Calories
Custard:		
(Morton)	20-oz. pie	1218
(Mrs. Smith's)	8" pie	1592
COCONUT PUDDING MIX:		
Cream, instant (Jell-O)	½ cup	188
Toasted, instant (Royal)	½ cup	184
COD:		
Raw, whole	1 lb.	110
Dehydrated	4 oz.	425
Frozen (Gorton)	1-lb. pkg.	351
COFFEE:		
*Regular (Maxwell House)	¾ cup	2
Instant *Nescafé*	1 rounded tsp.	4
*Decaffeinated, *Sanka,* instant	¾ cup	4
Freeze-dried, *Taster's Choice*	1 rounded tsp.	4
COFFEE CAKE:		
(Drake's) large	11-oz. cake	1230
Blueberry ring (Sara Lee)	1 oz.	108
Danish, apple (Morton)	13.5-oz. cake	1130
Danish, apple (Sara Lee)	1 oz.	84
Danish, cherry (Sara Lee)	1 oz.	75
Danish pecan twist (Morton)	12-oz. cake	1369
Lemon ring (Drake's)	13-oz. cake	1028
Melt-A-Way (Morton)	13-oz. cake	1511
Pecan ring (Drake's)	13-oz. cake	1109
Raspberry ring (Drake's)	13-oz. cake	1028
*COFFEE CAKE MIX (Aunt Jemima)	1 cake	1456
COLA SOFT DRINK:		
Sweetened:		
(Canada Dry) Jamaica	6 fl. oz.	75
(Clicquot Club) (Cott) (Mission)	6 fl. oz.	83
Coca-Cola	6 fl. oz.	73
(Dr. Brown's) (Hoffman) (Nedick's)		
(Royal Crown) (Waldbaum)		
(Yukon Club)	6 fl. oz.	81
(Key Food) regular	6 fl. oz.	77

*Prepared as Package Directs

Food and Description	Measure or Quantity	Calories
(Key Food) cherry	6 fl. oz.	75
Mr. Cola	6 fl. oz.	79
Pepsi-Cola	6 fl. oz.	78
RC with a twist (Royal Crown)	6 fl. oz.	74
(Shasta)	6 fl. oz.	76
(White Rock)	6 fl. oz.	80
Low calorie:		
(Canada Dry); (No-Cal); (Shasta);		
Tab	6 fl. oz.	<1
(Clicquot Club) (Cott) (Mission)	6 fl. oz.	2
Diet Pepsi-Cola, sugar-free	6 fl. oz.	<1
Diet Rite, sugar-free	6 fl. oz.	<1
(Dr. Brown's) (Hoffman) (Key		
Food) (Waldbaum) (Yukon Club)	6 fl. oz.	1
COLD DUCK WINE (Italian Swiss		
Colony—Private Stock) 12% alcohol	3 fl. oz.	75
COLLARDS:		
Raw, leaves and stems	1 lb.	181
Frozen, chopped (Birds Eye)	10-oz. pkg.	87
COLLINS MIX (Bar-Tender's)	1 serving	70
CONCENTRATE (Kellogg's)	1 oz.	108
CONCORD WINE (Mogen David)		
12% alcohol	3 fl. oz.	120
CONSOMME MADRILENE		
(Crosse & Blackwell)	1 can	66
COOKIE:		
Almond crescent (Nabisco)	1 piece	34
Almond toast, Mandel (Stella		
D'oro)	1 piece	49
Angelica Goodies (Stella D'oro)	1 piece	100
Anginetti (Stella D'oro)	1 piece	28
Animal cracker:		
(Nabisco) *Barnum's*	1 piece	12
(Sunshine)	1 piece	10
Anisette sponge (Stella D'oro)	1 piece	39

*Prepared as Package Directs

Food and Description	Measure or Quantity *	Calories
Anisette toast (Stella D'oro)	1 piece	39
Applesauce (Sunshine)	1 piece	86
Arrowroot (Sunshine)	1 piece	16
Assortment:		
(Stella D'oro) *Lady Stella*	1 piece	37
(Sunshine) *Lady Joan*	1 piece	42
Aunt Sally (Sunshine)	1 piece	96
Bana-Bee (Nabisco)	1¾-oz. pkg.	253
Big Treat (Sunshine)	1 piece	153
Bordeaux (Pepperidge Farm)	1 piece	36
Breakfast Treats (Stella D'oro)	1 piece	99
Brown edge wafers (Nabisco)	1 piece	28
Brownie:		
(Drake's) Junior	⅔-oz. cake	80
(Hostess) 2 to pkg.	1 piece	100
(Tastykake)	2¼-oz. pkg.	242
Chocolate nut (Pepperidge Farm)	1 piece	54
Peanut butter (Tastykake)	1¾-oz. pkg.	239
Pecan fudge (Keebler)	1 piece	115
Brussels (Pepperidge Farm)	1 piece	42
Butter (Nabisco) (Sunshine)	1 piece	23
Buttercup (Keebler)	1 piece	24
Butterscotch Fudgies (Tastykake)	1¾-oz. pkg.	251
Capri (Pepperidge Farm)	1 piece	82
Cardiff (Pepperidge Farm)	1 piece	18
Cherry Coolers (Sunshine)	1 piece	29
Chinese almond (Stella D'oro)	1 piece	178
Chocolate or chocolate-covered:		
Como (Stella D'oro)	1 piece	155
Creme (Wise)	1 piece	32
Peanut bars (Nabisco) *Ideal*	1 piece	94
Pinwheels (Nabisco)	1 piece	139
Snaps (Nabisco)	1 piece	18
Snaps (Sunshine)	1 piece	14
Wafers (Nabisco) *Famous*	1 piece	28
Chocolate chip:		
(Keebler) old fashioned	1 piece	80
(Nabisco)	1 piece	33
(Nabisco) *Chips Ahoy*	1 piece	51
(Nabisco) *Family Favorites*	1 piece	33
(Nabisco) snaps	1 piece	21
(Pepperidge Farm)	1 piece	52

*Prepared as Package Directs

Food and Description	Measure or Quantity	Calories
(Sunshine) *Chip-A-Roos*	1 piece	63
(Tastykake) *Choc-O-Chip*	1¾-oz. pkg.	283
Cinnamon:		
Crisp (Keebler)	1 piece	17
Spice, vanilla sandwich		
(Nabisco) *Crinkles*	1⅝-oz. pkg.	228
Sugar (Pepperidge Farm)	1 piece	52
Toast (Sunshine)	1 piece	13
Coconut:		
Bar (Nabisco)	1 piece	45
Bar (Sunshine)	1 piece	47
Chocolate chip (Nabisco)	1 piece	77
Chocolate chip (Sunshine)	1 piece	80
Chocolate drop (Keebler)	1 piece	75
Coconut Kiss (Tastykake)	1¾-oz. pkg.	318
Jumble (Drake's)	1 piece	70
Commodore (Keebler)	1 piece	65
Como Delight (Stella D'oro)	1 piece	153
Cowboys and Indians (Nabisco)	1 piece	10
Cream Lunch (Sunshine)	1 piece	45
Creme Wafer Stick (Dutch Twin)	1 piece	36
Creme Wafer Stick (Nabisco)	1 piece	50
Cup Custard (Sunshine)	1 piece	70
Devil's Food Cake (Nabisco)	1 piece	49
Dixie Vanilla (Sunshine)	1 piece	60
Dresden (Pepperidge Farm)	1 piece	83
Egg Jumbo (Stella D'oro)	1 piece	40
Fig bar:		
(Keebler)	1 piece	71
(Nabisco) *Fig Newtons*	1 piece	57
(Sunshine)	1 piece	45
Fortune (Chun King)	1 piece	31
Fruit, iced (Nabisco)	1 piece	71
Fudge:		
(Sunshine)	1 piece	72
Chip (Pepperidge Farm)	1 piece	51
Fudge Stripes (Keebler)	1 piece	57
Gingersnap:		
(Keebler)	1 piece	24
(Nabisco) old fashioned	1 piece	29
(Sunshine)	1 piece	24
Zu Zu (Nabisco)	1 piece	16

*Prepared as Package Directs

Food and Description	Measure or Quantity	Calories
Golden Bars (Stella D'oro)	1 piece	123
Golden Fruit (Sunshine)	1 piece	61
Hermit bar, frosted (Tastykake)	2-oz. pkg.	321
Home Plate (Keebler)	1 piece	58
Hydrox (Sunshine)	1 piece	48
Jan Hagel (Keebler)	1 piece	44
Keebies (Keebler)	1 piece	51
Lemon:		
(Sunshine)	1 piece	76
Jumble rings (Nabisco)	1 piece	68
Lemon Coolers (Sunshine)	1 piece	29
Nut crunch (Pepperidge Farm)	1 piece	57
Snaps (Nabisco)	1 piece	17
Lido (Pepperidge Farm)	1 piece	91
Lisbon (Pepperidge Farm)	1 piece	28
Macaroon:		
Almond (Tastykake)	2-oz. pkg.	336
Coconut (Nabisco) *Bake Shop*	1 piece	87
Sandwich (Nabisco)	1 piece	71
Margherite (Stella D'oro)	1 piece	73
Marquisette (Pepperidge Farm)	1 piece	45
Marshmallow:		
Fancy Crests (Nabisco)	1 piece	53
Mallowmars (Nabisco)	1 piece	60
Mallo Puff (Sunshine)	1 piece	63
Minarets (Nabisco)	1 piece	46
Puffs (Nabisco)	1 piece	94
Sandwich (Nabisco)	1 piece	32
Twirls (Nabisco)	1 piece	133
Milano (Pepperidge Farm)	1 piece	62
Milano, mint (Pepperidge Farm)	1 piece	76
Mint sandwich (Nabisco) *Mystic*	1 piece	88
Molasses & Spice (Sunshine)	1 piece	67
Naples (Pepperidge Farm)	1 piece	33
Nassau (Pepperidge Farm)	1 piece	83
Oatmeal:		
(Keebler) old fashioned	1 piece	79
(Nabisco)	1 piece	82
(Sunshine)	1 piece	58
Iced (Sunshine)	1 piece	69
Irish (Pepperidge Farm)	1 piece	50
Peanut butter (Sunshine)	1 piece	79

*Prepared as Package Directs

Food and Description	Measure or Quantity	Calories
Raisin (Nabisco) *Bake Shop*	1 piece	77
Raisin (Pepperidge Farm)	1 piece	55
Raisin bar (Tastykake)	2¼-oz pkg.	298
Old Country Treats (Stella D'oro)	1 piece	64
Orleans (Pepperidge Farm)	1 piece	30
Peach-apricot pastry (Stella D'oro)	1 piece	99
Peanut & peanut butter:		
Bars, cocoa-covered (Nabisco)		
Crowns	1 piece	92
Caramel logs (Nabisco) *Heydays*	1 piece	122
Creme patties (Nabisco)	1 piece	34
Creme patties, cocoa-covered		
(Nabisco) *Fancy*	1 piece	60
Patties (Sunshine)	1 piece	33
Sandwich (Nabisco) *Nutter*		
Butter	1 piece	69
Pecan Sandies (Keebler)	1 piece	85
Penguins (Keebler)	1 piece	111
Pirouette (Pepperidge Farm)	1 piece	38
Pitter Patter (Keebler)	1 piece	84
Pizzelle, Carolines (Stella D'oro)	1 piece	49
Raisin, fruit biscuit (Nabisco)	1 piece	58
Rich 'n Chips (Keebler)	1 piece	73
Rochelle (Pepperidge Farm)	1 piece	81
Sandwich, creme:		
Cameo (Nabisco)	1 piece	68
Chocolate chip (Nabisco)	1 piece	73
Chocolate fudge:		
(Keebler)	1 piece	99
(Nabisco) *Cookie Break*	1 piece	52
Orbit (Sunshine)	1 piece	51
Oreo (Nabisco)	1 piece	51
Oreo & Swiss (Nabisco)	1 piece	51
Pride (Nabisco)	1 piece	55
Social Tea (Nabisco)	1 piece	51
Swiss (Nabisco)	1 piece	52
(Tom Houston)	1 piece	74
Vanilla (Keebler)	1 piece	82
Vanilla (Nabisco)	1 piece	52
Vienna Finger (Sunshine)	1 piece	71
Sesame, Regina (Stella D'oro)	1 piece	51

*Prepared as Package Directs

Shortbread or shortcake:
  (Nabisco) *Dandy* — 1 piece — 46
  (Pepperidge Farm) — 1 piece — 72
  Lorna Doone (Nabisco) — 1 piece — 37
  Pecan (Nabisco) — 1 piece — 80
  Scotties (Sunshine) — 1 piece — 39
  Striped (Nabisco) — 1 piece — 50
  Vanilla (Tastykake) — 2¼-oz. pkg. — 352
Social Tea biscuit (Nabisco) — 1 piece — 21
Spiced wafers (Nabisco) — 1 piece — 41
Sprinkles (Sunshine) — 1 piece — 57
Sugar cookies:
  (Keebler) old fashioned — 1 piece — 78
  (Pepperidge Farm) — 1 piece — 51
  (Sunshine) — 1 piece — 86
  Brown (Nabisco) *Family Favorite* — 1 piece — 25
  Brown (Pepperidge Farm) — 1 piece — 48
  Rings (Nabisco) — 1 piece — 69
Sugar wafer:
  (Nabisco) *Biscos* — 1 piece — 19
  (Sunshine) — 1 piece — 43
  Krisp Kreem (Keebler) — 1 piece — 31
  Lemon (Sunshine) — 1 piece — 44
Swedish Kreme (Keebler) — 1 piece — 98
Tahiti (Pepperidge Farm) — 1 piece — 84
Toy (Sunshine) — 1 piece — 13
Vanilla creme (Wise) — 1 piece — 33
Vanilla snap (Nabisco) — 1 piece — 13
Vanilla wafer:
  (Keebler) — 1 piece — 19
  (Nabisco) *Nilla* — 1 piece — 18
  (Sunshine) small — 1 piece — 15
Venice (Pepperidge Farm) — 1 piece — 57
Waffle creme (Dutch Twin) — 1 piece — 44
Waffle creme (Nabisco) *Biscos* — 1 piece — 42
Yum Yums (Sunshine) — 1 piece — 83

COOKIE, DIETETIC:
Apple pastry (Stella D'oro) — 1 piece — 94
Assorted (Estee) — 1 piece — 31
Chocolate & vanilla wafer (Estee) — 1 piece — 27
Vanilla filled wafer (Estee) — 1 piece — 25

*Prepared as Package Directs

Food and Description	Measure or Quantity	Calories
COOKIE DOUGH, refrigerated (Pillsbury):		
Brownie	1 oz.	110
Chocolate chip	1 oz.	116
Peanut butter	1 oz.	129
COOKIE MIX:		
Brownie:		
*"Cake like," family size (Duncan Hines)	1 pan	3552
*Fudge, chewy, family size (Duncan Hines)	1 pan	3408
Fudge (Pillsbury)	1 oz.	125
*German chocolate (Betty Crocker)	1½" sq.	70
Toll House (Nestlé's)	1 oz.	132
COOL 'n CREAMY (Birds Eye)	½ cup	172
CORN:		
Raw, in husk	1 lb.	157
Raw, husk removed	1 lb.	240
Canned, regular pack:		
Vacuum pack (Green Giant)	12-oz. can	273
Country style (Green Giant)	8.5-oz. can	184
Cream style (Green Giant)	8.5-oz. can	212
Canned, dietetic pack (Blue Boy)	4 oz.	78
Frozen:		
(Birds Eye)	1 ear	98
& peppers, *Mexicorn*	10-oz. pkg.	281
Cream style (Green Giant)	10-oz. pkg.	204
In butter sauce (Niblets)	10-oz. pkg.	284
Kernel (Birds Eye)	½ cup	77
CORNBREAD (Aunt Jemima) corn sticks	3 pieces	134
CORNBREAD MIX:		
*(Aunt Jemima)	1 cornbread	1356
(Pillsbury) *Ballard*	1 oz.	103
CORN CHEX	1 oz.	107

*Prepared as Package Directs

[44]

Food and Description	Measure or Quantity	Calories
CORNED BEEF:		
Uncooked	1 lb.	1329
Canned (Armour Star)	12-oz. can	967
Packaged (Vienna)	1 oz.	68
CORNED BEEF HASH:		
(Armour Star)	15½-oz. can	831
(Austex)	15-oz. can	769
(Wilson)	15½-oz. can	792
CORNED BEEF SPREAD (Under-wood)	4½-oz. can	248
CORN FLAKES:		
Country (General Mills)	1 oz.	111
(Kellogg's) (Ralston)	1 oz.	108
(Van Brode)	1 oz.	106
CORN FRITTER (Mrs. Paul's)	12-oz. pkg.	846
CORNMEAL MIX (Aunt Jemima/Quaker)	¼ cup	96
CORN SOUFFLE (Stouffer's)	12-oz. pkg.	492
CORNSTARCH (Argo) (Kingsford's) (Duryea's)	1 T.	34
CORN TOTAL (General Mills)	1 oz.	111
COUNT CHOCULA (General Mills)	1 oz.	106
CRAB:		
Steamed, whole	1 lb.	202
Steamed, meat only	1 lb.	422
Canned:		
(Del Monte) Alaska King	7½-oz. can	202
(Icy Point) (Pillar Rock)	7½-oz. can	215
Frozen (Ship Ahoy) King Crab	8-oz. pkg.	211
CRAB APPLE	1 lb.	284
CRAB CAKE (Mrs. Paul's)	10-oz. pkg.	632

*Prepared as Package Directs

Food and Description	Measure or Quantity	Calories
CRAB COCKTAIL (Sau-Sea)	4-oz. jar	80
CRAB, DEVILED (Mrs. Paul's)	4 oz.	230
CRAB NEWBURG (Stouffer's)	12-oz. pkg.	562
CRAB SOUP (Crosse & Blackwell)	1 can	118
CRACKER:		
American Harvest (Nabisco)	1 piece	16
Arrowroot biscuit (Nabisco)	1 piece	22
Bacon flavored thins (Nabisco)	1 piece	11
Bacon Nips	1 oz.	147
Bacon rinds (Wonder)	1 oz.	146
Bacon toast (Keebler)	1 piece	15
Bugles (General Mills)	15 pieces	81
Butter thins (Nabisco)	1 piece	15
Cheese flavored:		
Cheese 'n Cracker (Kraft)	4 crackers & ¾ oz. cheese	138
Cheese Nips (Nabisco)	1 piece	5
Chee·Tos	1 oz.	156
Cheez Doodles (Old London)	1⅛-oz. bag	170
Cheez-Its (Sunshine)	1 piece	6
Cheez Waffles (Old London)	1 piece	11
Che-zo (Keebler)	1 piece	5
Combo Cheez (Austin's)	1 piece	26
Ritz (Nabisco)	1 piece	17
Shapies (Nabisco)	1 piece	9
Thins (Pepperidge Farm)	2 pieces	23
Thins, dietetic (Estee)	1 piece	6
Tid-Bit (Nabisco)	1 piece	4
Toast (Keebler)	1 piece	16
Twists (Nalley)	1 oz.	155
Twists (Wonder)	1 oz.	154
Chicken in a Biskit (Nabisco)	1 piece	10
Chippers (Nabisco)	1 piece	14
Chipsters (Nabisco)	1 piece	2
Clam flavored crisps (Snow)	1 oz.	147
Club (Keebler)	1 piece	15
Corn Capers (Wonder)	1 oz.	158
Corn cheeze (Tom Houston)	10 pieces	29

*Prepared as Package Directs

Food and Description	Measure or Quantity	Calories
Corn chips:		
Cornetts	1 oz.	153
Fritos	1 oz.	159
Korkers (Nabisco)	1 piece	8
(Old London)	1¾-oz. bag	263
(Wise)	1¾-oz. bag	276
(Wonder)	1 oz.	162
Barbecue (Wise)	1¾-oz. bag	274
Corn Diggers (Nabisco)	1 piece	4
Crown Pilot (Nabisco)	1 piece	73
Dipsy Doodles (Old London)	1¾-oz. bag	276
Doo Dads (Nabisco)	1 piece	2
Escort (Nabisco)	1 piece	20
Flings (Nabisco)	1 piece	11
Goldfish (Pepperidge Farm):		
Cheddar cheese	10 pieces	28
Lightly salted	10 pieces	28
Parmesan cheese	10 pieces	28
Pizza	10 pieces	29
Pretzel	10 pieces	29
Onion	10 pieces	28
Sesame garlic	10 pieces	29
Graham:		
(Nabisco)	1 piece	30
Chocolate or cocoa-covered:		
(Keebler) Deluxe	1 piece	42
(Nabisco)	1 piece	55
(Nabisco) Fancy	1 piece	68
(Nabisco) Pantry	1 piece	62
Sweet-Tooth (Sunshine)	1 piece	45
Sugar-honey coated (Nabisco)		
Honey Maid	1 piece	30
Hi-Ho (Sunshine)	1 piece	18
Milk lunch (Nabisco) Royal Lunch	1 piece	55
Munchos	1 oz.	148
Onion flavored:		
Crisps (Snow)	1 oz.	157
French (Nabisco)	1 piece	12
Funyuns (Frito-Lay)	1 oz.	141
Meal Mates (Nabisco)	1 piece	19
Onyums (General Mills)	30 pieces	79
Rings (Old London)	½-oz. bag	68

*Prepared as Package Directs

Food and Description	Measure or Quantity	Calories
Rings (Wise)	½-oz. bag	65
Rings (Wonder)	1 oz.	133
Thins (Pepperidge Farm)	1 piece	12
Toast (Keebler)	1 piece	18
OTC (Original Trenton Cracker)	1 piece	23
Oyster:		
(Keebler)	1 piece	2
(Nabisco) (Sunshine)	1 piece	3
Peanut butter 'n cheez crackers		
(Kraft)	4 crackers & ¾ oz. peanut butter	191
Peanut butter sandwich:		
Cheese crackers (Wise)	1 piece	30
Toasted crackers (Wise)	1 piece	30
Pizza Spins (General Mills)	32 pieces	72
Pizza Wheels (Wise)	¾-oz. bag	90
Potato crisps (General Mills)	16 pieces	78
Ritz, plain (Nabisco)	1 piece	16
Rye thins (Pepperidge Farm)	1 piece	10
Rye toast (Keebler)	1 piece	17
Rye wafers (Nabisco) *Meal Mates*	1 piece	19
Ry-Krisp:		
Seasoned	1 whole cracker	27
Traditional	1 whole cracker	23
Saltine:		
Flavor-Kist, any kind	1 piece	12
Krispy (Sunshine)	1 piece	11
Premium (Nabisco)	1 piece	12
Zesta (Keebler)	1 piece	12
Sea toast (Keebler)	1 piece	62
Sesame:		
(Sunshine) *La Lanne*	1 piece	15
Buttery flavored (Nabisco)	1 piece	16
Wafer (Keebler)	1 piece	16
Wafer (Nabisco) *Meal Mates*	1 piece	21
Sesa Wheat (Austin's)	1 piece	34
Sip 'n Chips (Nabisco)	1 piece	9
Sociables (Nabisco)	1 piece	10
Soda:		
(Nabisco) *Premium*	1 piece	12
(Sunshine)	1 piece	20
Soya (Sunshine) *La Lanne*	1 piece	16

*Prepared as Package Directs

Food and Description	Measure or Quantity	Calories
Star Lites (Wise)	1 cup	63
Swedish rye wafer (Keebler)	1 piece	5
Taco tortilla chips (Wonder)	1 oz.	144
Tortilla chips (Frito-Lay) *Doritos*	1 oz.	137
Tortilla chips (Old London)	1½-oz. bag	207
Tortilla chips (Wonder)	1 oz.	148
Town House	1 piece	18
Triangle Thins (Nabisco)	1 piece	8
Triscuit (Nabisco)	1 piece	21
Twigs (Nabisco)	1 piece	14
Uneeda Biscuit (Nabisco)	1 piece	22
Wafer-ets (Hol-Grain):		
Rice	1 piece	12
Wheat	1 piece	7
Waldorf, low salt (Keebler)	1 piece	14
Waverly wafer (Nabisco)	1 piece	18
Wheat chips (General Mills)	12 pieces	73
Wheat thins (Nabisco)	1 piece	9
Wheat toast (Keebler)	1 piece	16
Whistles (General Mills)	17 pieces	71
White thins (Pepperidge Farm)	1 piece	12
Whole-wheat, natural (Froumine)	1 piece	46

CRACKER CRUMBS, graham:

(Keebler)	3 oz.	368
(Nabisco)	9″ pie shell	563

CRACKER MEAL:

(Keebler) Zesty	3 oz.	363
Unsalted (Nabisco)	1 cup	319

CRANAPPLE (Ocean Spray):

Regular	½ cup	94
Low calorie	½ cup	19

CRANBERRY, fresh (Ocean Spray)   1 lb.   236

CRANBERRY JUICE COCKTAIL
  (Ocean Spray):

Regular	½ cup	83
Low calorie	½ cup	24

*Prepared as Package Directs

Food and Description	Measure or Quantity	Calories
CRANBERRY SAUCE:		
Jellied (Ocean Spray)	4 oz.	184
Whole berry (Ocean Spray)	4 oz.	191
CRANPRUNE (Ocean Spray)	½ cup	82
CRAYFISH, raw, in shell	1 lb.	39
CREAM:		
Half & half, 10.5% fat (Sealtest)	½ pt.	296
Light, 18% fat (Sealtest)	½ pt.	448
Heavy, whipping, 36% fat (Sealtest)	½ pt.	832
Sour:		
(Breakstone)	8-oz. container	464
Half & half (Sealtest)	½ pt.	320
Imitation, *Sour Treat* (Delite)	½ pt.	400
***CREAM OF RICE**	4 oz.	82
CREAM or CREME SOFT DRINK:		
Sweetened:		
(Canada Dry) vanilla	6 fl. oz.	97
(Clicquot Club) (Cott) (Mission)	6 fl. oz.	88
(Dr. Brown's) (Key Food)		
(Nedick's) (Shasta) (Waldbaum)	6 fl. oz.	84
(Fanta)	6 fl. oz.	94
(Hoffman) (Yukon Club)	6 fl. oz.	85
Low calorie:		
(Clicquot Club) (Cott) (Mission)	6 fl. oz.	3
(Dr. Brown's) (Hoffman) (Key		
Food) (Waldbaum) (Yukon Club)	6 fl. oz.	1
(No-Cal)	6 fl. oz.	2
(Shasta)	6 fl. oz.	<1
CREAM SUBSTITUTE:		
Coffee-mate (Carnation)	1 packet	17
Cremora (Borden); *Pream*	1 tsp.	11
CREAM OF WHEAT:		
Instant or quick	1 oz.	99
Regular	1 oz.	102
CREME DE CACAO LIQUEUR,		
(Bols) 54 proof	1 fl. oz.	101

*Prepared as Package Directs

Food and Description	Measure or Quantity	Calories
CREME DE MENTHE LIQUEUR (Garnier) 60 proof	1 fl. oz.	110
CRESS, GARDEN, raw, whole	1 lb.	103
CUCUMBER, fresh, whole	1 lb.	64
CUPCAKE:		
Chocolate (Tastykake)	1 cupcake	192
Chocolate, cream filled (Drake's)	1 cupcake	187
Devil's food cake (Hostess) 12 to pkg.	1 cupcake	122
Orange (Hostess) 12 to pkg.	1 cupcake	133
Raisin Snack (Drake's)	2¼-oz. cake	233
CUPCAKE MIX (Flako)	1 pkg.	1616
CURACAO LIQUEUR (Hiram Walker) 60 proof	1 fl. oz.	96
CURRANT:		
Fresh, whole	1 lb.	220
Dried (Del Monte)	½ cup	205
CURRY POWDER (Crosse & Blackwell)	1 T.	21
CUSTARD, chilled (Sealtest)	4 oz.	149
CUSTARD PUDDING MIX (Lynden Farms)	4-oz. pkg.	441

D

Food and Description	Measure or Quantity	Calories
DAIQUIRI COCKTAIL:		
Cocktail (Hiram Walker) 52.5 proof	3 fl. oz.	177
Cocktail (National Distillers) *Duet,* 12½% alcohol	8 fl. oz.	280
Mix (Bar-Tender's)	1 serving	70
DANDELION GREENS	1 lb.	204

*Prepared as Package Directs

Food and Description	Measure or Quantity	Calories
DANISH-STYLE VEGETABLES		
(Birds Eye)	10-oz. pkg.	276
DATE, dry:		
Chopped (Dromedary)	1 cup	493
Pitted (Dromedary)	1 cup	470
DESSERT CUP (Del Monte)	5-oz. container	173
DEVIL DOG (Drake's)	1.6-oz. cake	176
DEVIL'S FOOD CAKE (Pepperidge Farm)	1 cake	1956
DEVIL'S FOOD CAKE MIX:		
*(Duncan Hines)	1 cake	2460
*(Swans Down)	1 cake	2208
Red Devil (Pillsbury)	1 oz.	119
DING DONG (Hostess) 12 to pkg.	1 piece	162
DIP:		
Bacon & horseradish:		
(Breakstone)	2 T.	62
(Kraft) *Teez*	1 oz.	57
Blue cheese (Sealtest) *Dip 'n Dressing*	1 oz.	49
Clam:		
(Kraft) *Teez*	1 oz.	45
& lobster (Borden)	1 oz.	58
Jalapeño bean (Fritos)	1 oz.	37
Onion (Sealtest)	1 oz.	46
DIP MIX:		
Bacon-onion (Fritos)	1 pkg.	47
Bleu cheese (Fritos)	1 pkg.	48
Chili con queso (Fritos)	1 pkg.	72
Green onion (Fritos)	1 pkg.	49
Green onion (Lawry's)	1 pkg.	50
Guacamole (Lawry's)	1 pkg.	60
Toasted onion (Frito's)	1 pkg.	47
Toasted onion (Lawry's)	1 pkg.	48

*Prepared as Package Directs

DISTILLED LIQUOR:

80 proof	1 fl. oz.	65
86 proof	1 fl. oz.	70
90 proof	1 fl. oz.	74
94 proof	1 fl. oz.	77
100 proof	1 fl. oz.	83

DOUGHNUT:

(Hostess) 10 to pkg.	1 piece	139
Powdered (Morton)	1 piece	82

***DRAMBUIE* LIQUEUR,** 80 proof

(Hiram Walker)	1 fl. oz.	110

DR. BROWN'S CEL-RAY TONIC:

Regular	6 fl. oz.	66
Low calorie	6 fl. oz.	1

DR. PEPPER:

Regular	6 fl. oz.	71
Sugar free	6 fl. oz.	2

DUCK, raw, ready-to-cook	1 lb.	143

E

EGG, CHICKEN, raw:

Whole, medium	1 egg	71
Whole, large	1 egg	81
Whole, extra large	1 egg	94
Whole, jumbo	1 egg	105

EGG FOO YOUNG (Chun King)	12-oz. pkg.	240

EGG NOG:

(Borden) 4.7% fat	½ cup	132
(Meadow Gold) 6% fat	½ cup	164
(Sealtest) 8% butterfat	½ cup	192
With alcohol (Old Mr. Boston)		
30 proof	1 fl. oz.	83

EGGPLANT:

Fried sticks (Mrs. Paul's)	7-oz. pkg.	516
Parmesan (Mrs. Paul's)	11-oz. pkg.	632

*Prepared as Package Directs

Food and Description	Measure or Quantity	Calories
EGG ROLL:		
Chicken (Chun King)	½-oz. roll	28
Shrimp (Chun King)	½-oz. roll	24
***EGGSTRA** (Tillie Lewis)	1 large egg	42
ENCHILADA:		
Beef (Banquet)	2-lb. pkg.	1297
With rice (Swanson)	9⅝-oz. pkg.	378
ENCHILADA DINNER:		
Beef:		
(Banquet)	12-oz. dinner	467
(Patio) 5-compartment	13-oz. dinner	610
Cheese:		
(Banquet)	12½-oz. dinner	482
(Patio) 5-compartment	12-oz. dinner	380
ENCHILADA MIX (Lawry's)	1.6-oz. pkg.	144
ENDIVE, raw, curly	1 lb.	80

F

FARINA, cream (H-O)	1 cup	630
FAT, COOKING:		
Crisco; Fluffo	1 T.	103
Light Spry	1 T.	94
FIG:		
Fresh	1 lb.	363
Candied (Bama)	1 T.	37
Canned:		
(Del Monte)	½ cup	104
Unsweetened (Diet Delight)	½ cup	76
Dried (Del Monte)	1 cup	386
FIG JUICE, *RealFig*	½ cup	61
FILBERT or HAZELNUT, whole	1 lb.	1323
FISH CAKE, thins (Mrs. Paul's)	10-oz. pkg.	552

*Prepared as Package Directs

Food and Description	Measure or Quantity	Calories
FISH & CHIPS:		
(Gorton)	1-lb. pkg.	790
(Swanson)	5-oz. pkg.	268
FISH DINNER:		
With French fries (Swanson)	9¾-oz. dinner	429
With green beans & peach (Weight Watchers)	18-oz. dinner	266
With pineapple chunks (Weight Watchers)	9½-oz. luncheon	175
FISH FILLETS (Gorton)	8-oz. pkg.	480
FISH PUFFS (Gorton)	8-oz. pkg.	530
FISH STICK, breaded, fried (Mrs. Paul's)	14-oz. pkg.	756
FLOUNDER:		
Raw, whole	1 lb.	118
Frozen (Ship Ahoy)	1-lb. pkg.	316
FLOUR:		
Buckwheat, dark	1 cup	326
Rye, light	1 cup	361
Soybean	1 cup	329
Wheat:		
Aunt Jemima, self-rising	1 cup	384
Gold Medal (Betty Crocker):		
Regular	1 cup	483
Better-for-bread	1 cup	483
Self-rising	1 cup	476
Wondra	1 cup	483
Presto, self-rising	1 cup	381
Softasilk (Betty Crocker)	1 cup	412
FRANKFURTER or WIENER:		
(Armour Star) all meat	1.6-oz. frankfurter	155
(Oscar Mayer) all meat	1.6-oz. frankfurter	142
(Oscar Mayer) pure beef	1.6-oz. frankfurter	143
(Wilson) skinless, all meat	1.6-oz. frankfurter	140
Canned (Hormel)	12-oz. can	966

*Prepared as Package Directs

Food and Description	Measure or Quantity	Calories
FRANKS-n-BLANKETS (Durkee)	1 piece	45
FRENCH TOAST (Aunt Jemima)	1 slice	88
FRESCA	6 fl. oz.	<1
FROG LEGS	1 lb.	215
FROOT LOOPS (Kellogg's)	1 oz.	116
FROSTED RICE KRINKLES (Post)	1 oz.	111
FROSTED SHAKE (Borden)	9¼-fl.-oz. can	320
FROSTY O's (General Mills)	1 oz.	112
FROZEN DESSERT:		
Charlotte Freeze (Borden):		
Chocolate	1 pt.	450
Vanilla	1 pt.	414
Chocolate (SugarLo):		
4.6% fat, ice milk	1 pt.	420
10.8% fat, ice cream	1 pt.	591
Coffee (SugarLo):		
4% fat, ice milk	1 pt.	387
10% fat, ice cream	1 pt.	561
Strawberry (SugarLo):		
3.6% fat, ice milk	1 pt.	372
9% fat, ice cream	1 pt.	522
Vanilla-coated (SugarLo):		
Ice cream bar	2½-oz. bar	134
Ice milk bar	2½-oz. bar	111
FRUIT COCKTAIL:		
Canned, heavy syrup:		
(Hunt's)	½ cup	89
(Dole)	½ cup	94
Canned, unsweetened (Tillie Lewis)	½ cup	49
FRUIT CUP, solids & liquid (Del Monte):		
Fruit cocktail	5¼-oz. container	106

*Prepared as Package Directs

Food and Description	Measure or Quantity	Calories
Mixed fruit	5¼-oz. container	100
Peaches, diced	5¼-oz. container	107
Pineapple, in its own juice	4¼-oz. container	68
FRUITIFORT, cereal	1 oz.	111
FRUIT, MIXED:		
Dried (Del Monte)	1 cup	442
Quick thaw (Birds Eye)	½ cup	111
FRUIT SALAD:		
Chilled (Kraft)	4 oz.	57
Canned:		
(Del Monte) fruits for salad	½ cup	78
Unsweetened (S and W)		
Nutradiet	4 oz.	43
FUDGE CAKE MIX:		
Chocolate (Pillsbury)	1 oz.	120
*Marble (Duncan Hines)	1 cake	2424
Sour cream (Pillsbury)	1 oz.	118
FUDGE ICE BAR (Sealtest)	2½-fl.-oz. bar	91

G

Food and Description	Measure or Quantity	Calories
GARLIC, whole	2 oz.	68
GARLIC SPREAD (Lawry's)	1 T.	79
GATORADE	6 fl. oz.	53
GAZPACHO SOUP (Crosse & Blackwell)	13-oz. can	122
GEFILTE FISH:		
(Manischewitz) 1-lb. jar	1 piece	60
(Mother's) 1-lb. jar	1 piece	37
GELATIN (Knox)	1 envelope	28

*Prepared as Package Directs

Food and Description	Measure or Quantity	Calories
*GELATIN DESSERT POWDER:		
(Royal)	½ cup	82
(Jell-O)	½ cup	81
Dietetic (D-Zerta)	½ cup	8
GELATIN DRINK, orange (Knox)	1 envelope	30
GEL CUP (Del Monte):		
Lemon-lime with pineapple	5-oz. container	115
Orange with peaches	5-oz. container	107
Strawberry with peaches	5-oz. container	111
GERMAN DINNER (Swanson)	11-oz. dinner	405
GIN, SLOE (Garnier) 60 proof	1 fl. oz.	83
GINGER ALE, soft drink:		
Sweetened:		
(Canada Dry) (Clicquot Club) (Cott) (Fanta) (Mission) (White Rock) (Yukon Club)	6 fl. oz.	62
(Schweppes) (Shasta)	6 fl. oz.	66
Low calorie:		
(Canada Dry) (Clicquot Club) (Cott) (Mission) (No-Cal)	6 fl. oz.	2
(Dr. Brown's) (Hoffman) (Key Food) (Waldbaum) (Yukon Club)	6 fl. oz.	1
(Shasta)	6 fl. oz.	<1
*GINGERBREAD MIX		
(Dromedary)	2" x 2" piece	100
GINGER, CANDIED	1 oz.	96
GOOSE, raw, ready-to-cook	1 lb.	1172
GOOSEBERRY	1 lb.	177
GOULASH DINNER (Chef Boy-Ar-Dee)	7⅓-oz. pkg.	262

*Prepared as Package Directs

Food and Description	Measure or Quantity	Calories
GRANOLA:		
Sun Country, regular or almond	½ cup	253
Vita-Crunch:		
Regular	½ cup	295
Date	½ cup	284
Raisin	½ cup	289
Toasted almonds	½ cup	296
GRAPE, fresh, with skin:		
American type (slipskin)	1 lb.	196
European type (adherent skin)	1 lb.	278
GRAPEADE, chilled (Sealtest)	6 fl. oz.	96
GRAPE DRINK (Hi-C)	6 fl. oz.	88
*GRAPE DRINK MIX (Wyler's)	6 fl. oz.	64
GRAPE JELLY, low calorie (Kraft)	1 oz.	34
GRAPE JUICE:		
(Heinz)	5½-fl.-oz. can	130
*Frozen (Seneca)	½ cup	66
GRAPE-NUTS (Post)	1 oz.	104
GRAPE NUTS FLAKES (Post)	1 oz.	101
GRAPE SOFT DRINK:		
Sweetened:		
(Canada Dry)	6 fl. oz.	95
(Dr. Brown's) (Key Food)		
(Waldbaum)	6 fl. oz.	87
(Fanta)	6 fl. oz.	92
Grapette	6 fl. oz.	91
(Hoffman) (Nedick's) (Nehi)		
(Yukon Club)	6 fl. oz.	93
(Salute)	6 fl. oz.	102
(Shasta)	6 fl. oz.	88
(White Rock)	6 fl. oz.	89
(Yoo-Hoo)	6 fl. oz.	90
High-protein (Yoo-Hoo)	6 fl. oz.	114

*Prepared as Package Directs

Food and Description	Measure or Quantity	Calories
Low calorie:		
(Dr. Brown's) (Hoffman) (Key		
Food) (No-Cal) (Waldbaum)	6 fl. oz.	2
(Shasta) (Yukon Club)	6 fl. oz.	<1
GRAPEFRUIT:		
Fresh, pink & red:		
Seeded type	1 lb.	87
Seedless type	1 lb.	93
Fresh, white:		
Seeded type	1 lb.	84
Seedless type	1 lb.	87
Bottled, chilled (Kraft):		
Sweetened, sections	4 oz.	53
Unsweetened, sections	4 oz.	40
Canned:		
(Stokely-Van Camp)	½ cup	88
Unsweetened (Del Monte)		
(Tillie Lewis)	½ cup	45
GRAPEFRUIT JUICE:		
Chilled, sweetened (Kraft)	½ cup	60
Canned:		
Sweetened (Heinz)	5½-fl.-oz. can	73
Unsweetened (Heinz)	5½-fl.-oz. can	56
Frozen:		
*Sweetened (Minute Maid)		
(Snow Crop)	½ cup	57
Unsweetened (Minute Maid)		
(Snow Crop)	½ cup	50
GRAPEFRUIT PEEL (Liberty)	1 oz.	93
GRAVY:		
Brown with onion (Franco-American)	1 cup	96
Mushroom (B in B)	1 cup	176
Ready Gravy	1 cup	176
GRAVY MASTER	1 fl. oz.	49
GRAVY with MEAT:		
Sliced beef (Bunker Hill)	15-oz. can	716

*Prepared as Package Directs

Frozen:		
Giblet & sliced turkey (Banquet)	2-lb. pkg.	677
Sliced beef (Morton House)	6¼-oz. pkg.	189

GRAVY MIX:

Au jus (French's)	¾-oz. pkg.	44
Beef (Swiss Products)	1¼-oz. pkg.	107
Brown:		
(Durkee)	.8-oz. pkg.	59
(Lawry's)	1¼-oz. pkg.	136
(McCormick)	⅞-oz. pkg.	100
Chicken:		
(French's)	1¼-oz. pkg.	130
(Swiss)	⅞-oz. pkg.	75
Mushroom (Lawry's)	1.3-oz. pkg.	145
Onion (Durkee)	1-oz. pkg.	84

GRENADINE SYRUP (Giroux)

non-alcoholic	1 fl. oz.	100

GUINEA HEN, ready-to-cook

	1 lb.	594

H

HADDOCK:

Raw, whole	1 lb.	172
Smoked	4 oz.	117

HADDOCK DINNER:

(Banquet)	8.8-oz. dinner	424
(Weight Watchers)	18-oz. dinner	256

HALIBUT:

Atlantic & Pacific, raw, whole	1 lb.	268
California, raw, meat only	1 lb.	440

HAM:

Boiled (Hormel)	1 oz.	35
Canned:		
(Hormel)	1-lb. 8-oz. can	1152
(Oscar Mayer) *Jubilee*, boneless	1 lb.	826
Chopped or minced (Armour Star)	1 oz.	84

*Prepared as Package Directs

Food and Description	Measure or Quantity	Calories
Chopped (Hormel)	1 oz.	78
Deviled (Underwood)	4½-oz. can	438
HAM & CHEESE loaf (Oscar Mayer)	1-oz. slice	69
HAM DINNER:		
(Banquet)	10-oz. dinner	352
(Morton)	10-oz. dinner	429
(Swanson)	10¼-oz. dinner	366
HAWAIIAN DINNER MIX (Hunt's) *Skillet*	1-lb. pkg.	760
HAWAIIAN PUNCH (RJR Foods)	6 fl. oz.	82
HAWAIIAN-STYLE VEGETABLES (Birds Eye)	10-oz. pkg.	276
HEADCHEESE (Oscar Mayer)	1-oz. slice	52
HERRING:		
Raw, Atlantic, whole	1 lb.	407
Raw, Atlantic, meat only	1 lb.	444
Canned:		
Bismarck, drained (Vita)	5-oz. jar	273
In cream sauce (Vita)	8-oz. jar	397
Kippered	4 oz.	239
HICKORY NUT, whole	1 lb.	1068
HO-HO (Hostess) 10 to pkg.	1 piece	106
HOMINY GRITS (Quaker)	.8-oz. packet	80
HONEY	½ cup	496
HONEYDEW, whole	1 lb.	94
HORSERADISH:		
Raw, whole	1 lb.	288
Prepared cream style (Kraft)	1 oz.	9

*Prepared as Package Directs

I

ICE CREAM and FROZEN CUSTARD:

10% fat	1 pt.	514
12% fat	1 pt.	588
16% fat	1 pt.	658

ICE CREAM BAR (Sealtest) — 2½-fl.-oz. bar — 149

ICE CREAM CONE, cone only:

Assorted colors (Comet)	1 piece	19
Rolled sugar (Comet)	1 piece	49

ICE CREAM CUP, cup only:

(Comet)	1 piece	20
Pilot (Comet)	1 piece	19

ICE CREAM SANDWICH (Sealtest) — 3 fl. oz. — 173

ICE MILK:

(Borden) 3.5% fat	1 pt.	388
(Borden) *Lite-line*	1 pt.	396
Light n' Lively (Sealtest):		
Chocolate	1 pt.	420
Coffee	1 pt.	408
Strawberry	1 pt.	400
Vanilla	1 pt.	408

ICE CREAM BAR, chocolate-coated
(Sealtest) — 2½-fl.-oz. bar — 132

ICE STICK (Sealtest) — 3 fl. oz. — 70

INDIAN PUDDING (B & M) — ½ cup — 120

ITALIAN DINNER:

(Banquet)	11-oz. dinner	414
(Swanson)	13-oz. dinner	448

ITALIAN-STYLE VEGETABLES
(Birds Eye) — 10-oz. pkg. — 294

*Prepared as Package Directs

Food and Description	Measure or Quantity	Calories

J

JACK MACKEREL, meat only	1 lb.	648
JAM	1 oz.	77
JAPANESE-STYLE VEGETA-BLES (Birds Eye)	10-oz. pkg.	315
JELLY (Kraft)	1 oz.	74
JERUSALEM ARTICHOKE	1 lb.	207

K

KABOOM (General Mills)	1 oz.	109
KALE:		
Raw, leaves including stems	1 lb.	128
Frozen, chopped (Birds Eye)	½ cup	29
KARO, syrup:		
Dark corn	1 cup	973
Light corn	1 cup	967
Pancake & waffle	1 cup	967
KIDNEY, beef	1 lb.	588
KING VITAMIN (Quaker)	1 oz.	118
KIRSCH LIQUEUR (Garnier) 96 proof	1 fl. oz.	83
KIX, cereal	1 oz.	112
KNOCKWURST (Oscar Mayer) *Chubbies*	2.4 oz. link	210
KOHLRABI, whole	1 lb.	96
KOOL-AID (General Foods)	1 cup	98

*Prepared as Package Directs

Food and Description	Measure or Quantity	Calories
KRUMBLES (Kellogg's)	1 oz.	110
KUMQUAT, whole	1 lb.	274

L

Food and Description	Measure or Quantity	Calories
LAKE HERRING, whole	1 lb.	226
LAMB, raw:		
Loin, lean & fat	1 lb.	1146
Rib, lean & fat	1 lb.	1229
Leg, lean & fat	1 lb. (weighed with bone)	845
Shoulder, lean & fat	1 lb. (weighed with bone)	1082
LAMB STEW, canned (B & M)	1 cup	192
LARD	1 lb.	4091
LASAGNE:		
(Chef Boy-Ar-Dee)	40-oz. can	1116
(Buitoni)	56-oz. pkg.	1638
(Hunt's) *Skillet*	1-lb. 2-oz. pkg.	812
LEEKS, raw, whole	1 lb.	123
LEMON, whole	1 lb.	90
LEMONADE:		
Chilled (Sealtest)	½ cup	55
Frozen, sweetened (ReaLemon)	6-oz. can	414
***LEMON CAKE MIX,** pudding cake (Betty Crocker)	1 cake	1362
LEMON JUICE:		
(Sunkist)	1 lemon	11
Canned, plastic container *ReaLemon*	1 T.	3

*Prepared as Package Directs

Full strength, already reconstituted (Minute Maid) (Snow Crop)	½ cup	27

LEMON-LIME SOFT DRINK:
Sweetened:

(Dr. Brown's) (Hoffman) (Key Food) (Nedick's) (Waldbaum)	6 fl. oz.	74
(Salute)	6 fl. oz.	72
(Shasta)	6 fl. oz.	73
(White Rock)	6 fl. oz.	77

Low calorie:

(Hoffman) (Yukon Club)	6 fl. oz.	1
(Shasta)	6 fl. oz.	<1

LEMON PEEL, candied (Liberty)	1 oz.	93

LEMON PIE, cream, frozen:

(Morton)	14.4-oz. pie	1048
(Mrs. Smith's)	8″ pie	1364

LEMON PIE FILLING:

(Comstock)	½ cup	174
(Lucky Leaf)	8 oz.	412

LEMON PUDDING (Hunt's)	5-oz. can	175

LEMON PUDDING or PIE MIX:

*(Royal) including crust	9″ pie	1792
*Instant (Jell-O)	½ cup	178

LEMON SOFT DRINK:
Sweetened:

(Canada Dry) *Hi-Spot*	6 fl. oz.	72
(Clicquot Club) (Cott) (Mission)	6 fl. oz.	74
(Royal Crown)	6 fl. oz.	89

Low calorie:

(Canada Dry)	6 fl. oz.	1
(Clicquot Club) (Cott) (Mission)	6 fl. oz.	3
(No-Cal)	6 fl. oz.	2

*Prepared as Package Directs

Food and Description	Measure or Quantity	Calories
LENTIL:		
Whole, dry	½ lb.	771
Split, dry	½ lb.	782
LENTIL SOUP, with ham		
(Crosse & Blackwell)	13-oz. can	246
LETTUCE:		
Bibb, Boston	1 lb.	47
Grand Rapids, Romaine, Simpson	1 lb.	52
Iceberg, New York	1 lb.	56
LIEBFRAUMILCH WINE (Julius		
Kayser) Glockenspiel, 10% alcohol	3 fl. oz.	57
LIFE, cereal	1 oz.	107
LIKE, soft drink	6 fl. oz.	1
LIME	1 lime	15
LIMEADE (ReaLemon)	6-oz. can	414
LIME JUICE, plastic container,		
ReaLime	1 T.	2
LIME PIE (Banquet)	2½-oz. serving	204
LITCHI NUT, dried, whole	¼ lb.	145
LIVER, raw:		
Beef	1 lb.	635
Calf	1 lb.	635
Chicken	1 lb.	585
Hog	1 lb.	594
Lamb	1 lb.	617
LIVERWURST (Oscar Mayer)	.9-oz. slice	95
LIVERWURST SPREAD		
(Underwood)	1 T.	45

*Prepared as Package Directs

Food and Description	Measure or Quantity	Calories
LOBSTER, raw, whole	1 lb.	107
LOBSTER NEWBURG (Stouffer's)	11½-oz. pkg.	671
LOBSTER SOUP (Crosse & Blackwell)	13-oz. can	184
LOG CABIN, syrup	1 T.	46
LUNCHEON MEAT:		
All meat (Oscar Mayer)	1-oz. slice	98
Cocktail loaf (Oscar Mayer)	1-oz. slice	62
Luxury Loaf (Oscar Mayer)	1-oz. slice	40
Olive loaf (Oscar Mayer)	1-oz. slice	62
Pickle & pimento (Sugardale)	1-oz. slice	78
Spiced (Hormel)	1 oz.	70

M

Food and Description	Measure or Quantity	Calories
MACADAMIA NUT, shelled	4 oz.	784
MACARONI:		
Dry	1 oz.	105
20% Protein (Buitoni)	1 oz.	101
MACARONI & BEEF:		
Canned, tiny meatballs & sauce (Buitoni)	4 oz.	111
Frozen:		
(Banquet)	2-lb. pkg.	1092
With tomatoes (Stouffer's)	11½-oz. pkg.	410
MACARONI & CHEESE:		
(Heinz)	8¼-oz. can	231
Frozen:		
(Banquet)	20-oz. pkg.	742
(Morton)	8-oz. casserole	297
MACARONI DINNER:		
& cheese:		
*(Chef Boy-Ar-Dee)	4½-oz. pkg.	201

*Prepared as Package Directs

Food and Description	Measure or Quantity	Calories
(Banquet)	12-oz. dinner	342
Creole, with mushrooms (Heinz)	8¾-oz. can	169
MACARONI SALAD,		
canned (Nalley's)	4 oz.	203
MACKEREL:		
Raw, Atlantic, whole	1 lb.	468
Raw, Pacific, dressed	1 lb.	519
Salted	4 oz.	346
MADEIRA WINE (Leacock)		
19% alcohol	3 fl. oz.	120
MAI TAI COCKTAIL:		
(Lemon Hart) 48 proof	3 fl. oz.	180
(National Distillers)		
Duet, 12½% alcohol	8-fl.-oz. can	288
(Party Tyme) 12½% alcohol	2 fl. oz.	65
Dry mix (Bar-Tender's)	1 serving	69
Dry mix (Party Tyme)	1 serving	50
Liquid mix, canned (Party Tyme)	2 fl. oz.	44
MALTEX, cereal	1 oz.	109
MALT LIQUOR, *Country Club*	12 fl. oz.	183
MANDARIN ORANGE, CANNED:		
(Del Monte)	½ cup	77
(Diet Delight)	½ cup	31
(S and W) *Nutradiet*	4 oz.	31
MANGO, whole	1 lb.	201
MANHATTAN COCKTAIL:		
(Hiram Walker) 55 proof	3 fl. oz.	147
(National Distillers) *Duet,* 20%		
alcohol	8-fl.-oz. can	576
(Party Tyme) 20% alcohol	2 fl. oz.	74
Brandy (National Distillers)		
Duet, 20% alcohol	8-fl.-oz. can	560
Dry mix (Bar-Tender's)	1 serving	24

*Prepared as Package Directs

Food and Description	Measure or Quantity	Calories
MANICOTTI, with sauce (Buitoni)	4 oz.	150
MAPLE SYRUP (Cary's)	1 T.	63
MARBLE CAKE MIX (Betty Crocker)	1 cake	2472
MARGARINE	1 lb.	3266
MARGARINE, IMITATION (Mazola)	1 lb.	1610
MARGARINE, WHIPPED	1 cup	1094
MARGARITA COCKTAIL:		
(National Distillers) *Duet*, 12½% alcohol	8-fl.-oz. can	248
(Party Tyme) 12½% alcohol	2 fl. oz.	66
Dry mix (Bar-Tender's)	1 serving	70
Dry mix (Party Tyme)	1 serving	50
Liquid mix (Party Tyme)	2 fl. oz.	63
MARINADE MIX:		
(Adolph's)	.8-oz. pkg.	39
(Durkee)	.9-oz. pkg.	69
(Lawry's)	1.6-oz. pkg.	69
MARMALADE:		
Sweetened (Kraft)	1 oz.	78
Low calorie (Kraft)	1 oz.	35
MARTINI COCKTAIL:		
Gin:		
(Hiram Walker) 67.5 proof	3 fl. oz.	168
(National Distillers) *Duet*, 21% alcohol	8-fl.-oz. can	560
(Party Tyme) 24% alcohol	2 fl. oz.	82
Liquid mix (Party Tyme)	2 fl. oz.	12
Vodka:		
(Hiram Walker) 60 proof	3 fl. oz.	147
(National Distillers) *Duet*, 20% alcohol	8-fl.-oz. can	536
(Party Tyme) 21% alcohol	2 fl. oz.	72

*Prepared as Package Directs

Food and Description	Measure or Quantity	Calories
*MASA HARINA (Quaker)	2 tortillas	139
*MASA TRIGO (Quaker)	2 tortillas	149
MATZO:		
Regular (Manischewitz)	1 matzo	114
Tea (Goodman's)	1 matzo	70
Unsalted (Horowitz-Margareten)	1 matzo	135
MATZO MEAL (Manischewitz)	1 cup	438
MAYONNAISE:		
(Best Foods) Real; (Hellmann's)	1 T.	102
(Kraft)	1 T.	102
Saffola	1 T.	92
MAYPO, cereal	1 oz.	107
MEATBALL:		
In sauce (Prince)	3.7-oz. can	171
With gravy (Chef Boy-Ar-Dee)	15¼-oz. can	472
MEAT LOAF ENTREE (Swanson)	9-oz. pkg.	316
MEAT LOAF DINNER:		
(Banquet)	11-oz. dinner	420
(Morton) 3-course	1-lb. 1-oz. dinner	652
(Swanson) 3-course	16-oz. dinner	544
MEAT LOAF SEASONING MIX (Contadina)	3¾-oz. pkg.	363
MEAT, POTTED:		
(Armour Star)	3-oz. can	181
(Hormel)	3-oz. can	158
MELBA TOAST:		
Garlic, onion or plain (Keebler)	1 piece	9
Garlic, onion or sesame rounds (Old London)	1 piece	8

*Prepared as Package Directs

Food and Description	Measure or Quantity	Calories
Pumpernickel, wheat or white		
(Old London)	1 piece	15
Rye (Old London)	1 piece	14
Sesame (Keebler)	1 piece	11
MELON BALL, in syrup	½ cup	72
MEXICAN DINNER:		
Mix (Hunt's) *Skillet*	1-lb. 2-oz. pkg.	699
Frozen:		
Mexican style (Banquet)	16¼-oz. dinner	568
(Swanson)	18-oz. dinner	613
MEXICAN-STYLE VEGETA-		
BLES (Birds Eye)	10-oz. pkg.	432
MILK, CONDENSED, *Eagle Brand*	1 fl. oz.	125
MILK, DRY, nonfat, instant		
(Carnation)	1 cup	244
MILK, EVAPORATED (Borden)	14.5-oz. can	563
MILK, FRESH:		
Whole, 3.5% fat (Sealtest)	1 cup	151
Skim:		
Light n', Lively (Sealtest)	1 cup	114
Skim-line (Borden)	1 cup	99
Buttermilk:		
Light n' Lively (Sealtest)	1 cup	95
1% fat (Borden)	1 cup	107
Chocolate milk drink, fresh:		
With whole milk, 3.3% fat		
(Meadow Gold)	1 cup	200
With skim milk, 1% fat (Sealtest)	1 cup	158
MINCEMEAT:		
(Crosse & Blackwell)	1 cup	960
Condensed (None Such)	9-oz. pkg.	937
MINCE PIE:		
(Morton)	20-oz. pie	1482
(Mrs. Smith's)	8″ pie	2035

*Prepared as Package Directs

Food and Description	Measure or Quantity	Calories
MINESTRONE SOUP (Campbell)	1 can	164
MOLASSES:		
Dark (Brer Rabbit)	1 T.	53
Light (Brer Rabbit)	1 T.	60
Unsulphured (Grandma's)	1 T.	57
MORTADELLA	1 oz.	89
MRS. BUTTERWORTH'S SYRUP	1 T.	53
MUFFIN:		
Blueberry, frozen (Morton)	1.6-oz. muffin	116
Bran (Thomas') with raisins	1.9-oz. muffin	170
Corn (Thomas')	2-oz. muffin	194
English (Thomas')	2.1-oz. muffin	140
Scone (Wonder) *Raisin Round*	1 piece	149
MUFFIN MIX:		
*Blueberry (Betty Crocker)	2¾" muffin	118
*Corn (Flako)	1.3-oz. muffin	131
*Honey bran (Betty Crocker)	2¾" muffin	154
MUSHROOM:		
Raw, whole	½ lb.	62
Canned:		
(Oxford Royal)	4-oz. can	17
Sliced (B in B)	6-oz. can	50
Frozen, in butter sauce		
(Green Giant)	6-oz. pkg.	87
MUSHROOM SOUP, cream of		
(Heinz) *Great American*	1 cup	131
MUSHROOM SOUP MIX, cream		
of (Lipton) *Cup-a-Soup*	1 pkg.	86
MUSSEL, Atlantic & Pacific, raw	1 lb.	153
MUSTARD:		
Brown (French's) (Gulden's)	1 tsp.	6
Grey Poupon	1 tsp.	4
Yellow (Gulden's) (Heinz)	1 tsp.	5

*Prepared as Package Directs

MUSTARD GREENS:
Whole	1 lb.	98
Chopped (Birds Eye)	½ cup	19

N

NEAPOLITAN CREAM PIE:
(Morton)	14.4-oz. pie	1068
(Mrs. Smith's)	8" pie	1462

NECTARINE, whole — 1 lb. — 267

NOODLE, dry, 1½" strips — 1 oz. — 110

NOODLE & BEEF:
(Heinz)	8½-oz. can	171
(Nalley's)	2-lb. pkg.	735

NOODLE, CHOW MEIN (Hung's) — 1 oz. — 148

*****NOODLE DINNER,** Stroganoff mix
(Betty Crocker)	1 cup	500

NOODLE MIX:
*Almondine (Betty Crocker)	½ cup	213
*Romanoff, *Noodle-Roni*	4 oz.	179

NUT, mixed:
Dry roasted:
(Flavor House)	1 oz.	172
(Skippy)	1 oz.	181

Oil roasted:
With peanuts (Planters)	1 oz.	176
Without peanuts (Planters)	1 oz.	178

O

OAT FLAKES (Post) — 1 oz. — 107

OATMEAL:
Instant (Quaker)	1-oz. packet	107
Quick (H-O)	1 cup	267

*Prepared as Package Directs

Food and Description	Measure or Quantity	Calories
Regular:		
(Ralston)	1 oz.	103
*(Albers) old fashioned	1 cup	148
OCEAN PERCH:		
Raw, Atlantic, whole	1 lb.	124
Raw, Pacific, whole	1 lb.	116
Frozen (Gorton)	1-lb. pkg.	399
OCEAN PERCH MEALS, frozen:		
(Banquet)	8.8-oz. dinner	472
(Weight Watchers)	18-oz. dinner	307
OIL, salad or cooking:		
Corn (Mazola)	½ cup	981
Olive	½ cup	972
Peanut (Planters)	½ cup	1008
(Saff-o-life)	½ cup	972
Soybean	½ cup	972
OKRA:		
Raw, whole	1 lb.	140
Cut (Birds Eye)	½ cup	36
Whole (Birds Eye)	½ cup	27
OLD FASHIONED:		
Cocktail (Hiram Walker) 62 proof	3 fl. oz.	165
Mix (Bar-Tender's)	1 serving	20
OLIVE:		
Greek style, pitted	1 oz.	96
Green, pitted & drained:	1 oz.	33
Ripe	1 oz.	37
ONION:		
Raw, whole	1 lb.	157
Canned (Comstock-Greenwood)	4 oz.	33
Dehydrated, flakes	½ cup	112
Frozen:		
Chopped (Birds Eye)	¼ cup	11
Whole, small (Birds Eye)	½ cup	51
Small with cream sauce (Birds Eye)	9-oz. pkg.	396

*Prepared as Package Directs

Food and Description	Measure or Quantity	Calories
French-fried rings:		
(Durkee) O&C	3-oz. can	530
(Mrs. Paul's)	9-oz. pkg.	566
Pickled, cocktail (Crosse & Blackwell)	1 T.	1
ONION, GREEN, raw, whole	1 lb.	157
ONION SOUP (Hormel)	15-oz. can	144
ONION SOUP MIX (Lipton)		
Cup-a-Soup	1 pkg.	30
ONION, WELSH, whole	1 lb.	100
ORANGE:		
California Navel	1 lb.	157
California Valencia	1 lb.	174
Florida	1 lb.	158
ORANGEADE, chilled (Sealtest)	½ cup	64
ORANGE CAKE, frosted (Sara Lee)	2 oz.	206
ORANGE CREAM BAR (Sealtest)	2½-fl.-oz. bar	103
ORANGE DRINK (Hi-C)	6 fl. oz.	89
*****ORANGE-GRAPEFRUIT JUICE:**		
(Minute Maid) (Snow Crop)	½ cup	51
ORANGE ICE (Sealtest)	1 pt.	520
ORANGE JUICE:		
Fresh	½ cup	56
Chilled (Kraft)	½ cup	60
Canned, sweetened (Heinz)	5½-fl.-oz. can	91
Canned, unsweetened (Heinz)	5½-fl.-oz. can	71
Frozen:		
*(Lake Hamilton) (Nature's Best)	½ cup	58
*(Minute Maid) (Snow Crop)	½ cup	60

*Prepared as Package Directs

Food and Description	Measure or Quantity	Calories
ORANGE PEEL, candied (Liberty)	1 oz.	93
ORANGE PLUS (Birds Eye)	½ cup	67
ORANGE SOFT DRINK:		
Sweetened:		
(Canada Dry) *Orangette*	6 fl. oz.	94
(Clicquot Club) (Cott) (Mission)	6 fl. oz.	103
(Dr. Brown's) (Nedick's)		
(Waldbaum)	6 fl. oz.	91
(Fanta)	6 fl. oz.	92
(Hoffman)	6 fl. oz.	93
(Key Food)	6 fl. oz.	86
(Kirsch)	6 fl. oz.	88
(Nehi)	6 fl. oz.	100
(Salute)	6 fl. oz.	102
(Shasta) (Yukon Club)	6 fl. oz.	95
(White Rock)	6 fl. oz.	89
(Yoo-Hoo)	6 fl. oz.	90
High-protein (Yoo-Hoo)	6 fl. oz.	114
Low calorie:		
(Canada Dry) (Shasta)	6 fl. oz.	<1
(Clicquot Club) (Cott) (Mission)		
(No-Cal)	6 fl. oz.	2
(Dr. Brown's) (Hoffman) (Key		
Food) (Nedick's) (Waldbaum)		
(Yukon Club)	6 fl. oz.	1
ORIENTAL DINNER (Hunt's)		
Skillet	1-lb. 1-oz. pkg.	675
OVALTINE	1 oz.	111
OYSTER:		
Eastern, in shell	1 lb.	30
Eastern, meat only	1 lb.	300
Pacific & Western, meat only	1 lb.	412
Smoked, Japanese baby (Cresca)	3⅔-oz. can	222
OYSTER STEW (Campbell)	1 can	284

*Prepared as Package Directs

P

PANCAKE (Swanson)	6-oz. breakfast	463
PANCAKE & WAFFLE MIX:		
*Buckwheat (Aunt Jemima)	4″ pancake	61
Buttermilk (Pillsbury) *Hungry Jack*	1 oz.	98
Plain:		
*(Aunt Jemima) Complete	4″ pancake	59
*(Aunt Jemima) Easy Pour	4″ pancake	78
*(Aunt Jemima) Original	4″ pancake	59
PARISIAN-STYLE VEGETA-		
BLES (Birds Eye)	10-oz. pkg.	270
PARSLEY, fresh, whole	½ lb.	100
PARSNIP, whole	1 lb.	293
PASSION FRUIT, whole	1 lb.	212
PASTINAS, dry egg	1 oz.	109
PASTRAMI (Vienna)	1 oz.	57
PASTRY SHELL:		
Pot pie, bland (Keebler)	4″ shell	236
Frozen, tart (Pepperidge Farm)	3-oz. pie tart	276
PATE:		
Liver (Hormel)	1 oz.	78
Liver (Sell's)	1 oz.	90
PEA, GREEN:		
Raw, in pod	1 lb.	145
Raw, shelled	1 lb.	381
Canned:		
Early (Le Sueur)	8.5-oz. can	108
Sweet (Green Giant)	8.5-oz. can	108
Frozen:		
(Birds Eye)	10-oz. pkg.	210

*Prepared as Package Directs

Food and Description	Measure or Quantity	Calories
In butter sauce (Green Giant) *Le Sueur*	10-oz. pkg.	222
With cream sauce (Green Giant)	10-oz. pkg.	189
With sliced mushroom (Birds Eye)	10-oz. pkg.	198
PEA, MATURE SEED:		
Whole	1 lb.	1542
Split (Sinsheimer)	1 lb.	1584
PEA POD	1 lb.	228
PEA & CARROT:		
(Del Monte)	½ cup	46
Frozen:		
(Birds Eye)	10-oz. pkg.	165
In cream sauce (Green Giant)	10-oz. pkg.	168
PEA & CELERY (Birds Eye)	10-oz. pkg.	165
PEA & ONION, in butter sauce (Green Giant)	10-oz. pkg.	216
PEA & POTATO (Birds Eye)	1 pkg.	393
PEA SOUP, GREEN:		
Canned (Campbell)	1 can	262
Dry mix (Lipton) *Cup-a-Soup*	1 pkg.	127
PEA SOUP, SPLIT:		
(Manischewitz)	1 can	266
With smoked ham (Heinz) *Great American*	1 cup	186
PEACH:		
Fresh, whole	1 lb.	150
Canned:		
Heavy syrup (Hunt's)	½ cup	96
Spiced (Del Monte)	½ cup	96
Canned, dietetic:		
(Blue Boy)	4 oz.	32

*Prepared as Package Directs

Food and Description	Measure or Quantity	Calories
(Diet Delight) freestone	½ cup	64
(Tillie Lewis) Elberta	½ cup	40
Dried (Del Monte)	½ cup	199
Frozen (Birds Eye)	½ cup	87
PEACH NECTAR (Del Monte)	1 cup	140
PEACH PIE:		
(Morton)	20-oz. pie	1470
(Mrs. Smith's)	8" pie	1804
PEACH PIE FILLING:		
(Comstock)	½ cup	175
(Lucky Leaf)	8 oz.	300
PEACH TURNOVER (Pepperidge Farm)	1 turnover	323
PEANUT:		
Raw, in shell	1 lb.	1868
Roasted:		
Dry (Franklin)	1 oz.	163
Dry (Skippy)	1 oz.	180
Oil (Planters) cocktail	1 oz.	179
Spanish, dry roasted (Planters)	1 oz.	175
Spanish, oil roasted (Planters)	1 oz.	182
PEANUT BUTTER:		
(Bama) crunchy	1 T.	96
(Bama) smooth	1 T.	100
(Peter Pan)	1 T.	100
(Skippy)	1 T.	104
PEANUT SPREAD, diet (Peter Pan)	1 T.	100
PEAR:		
Fresh, whole	1 lb.	252
Canned:		
Juice pack (Libby's)	4 oz.	68
Heavy syrup (Hunt's)	½ cup	90
Canned, unsweetened (S and W)		
Nutradiet	2 halves	30
Dried (Del Monte)	½ cup	178

*Prepared as Package Directs

[80]

Food and Description	Measure or Quantity	Calories
PEAR NECTAR (Del Monte)	1 cup	140
PECAN:		
In shell	1 lb.	1652
Shelled	1 lb.	3116
Dry roasted (Planters)	1 oz.	206
PECAN PIE:		
(Morton)	20-oz. pie	2058
(Mrs. Smith's)	8″ pie	2580
PEPPER:		
Black	1 tsp.	4
Seasoned (Lawry's)	1.6-oz. pkg.	158
PEPPER, HOT CHILI:		
Green, raw	4 oz.	31
Red:		
Raw	4 oz.	105
Canned, drained (Ortega)	¼ cup	10
Dried (Chili Products)	1 oz.	88
PEPPER, STUFFED:		
(Holloway House)	7-oz. roll	178
Frozen, with veal (Weight Watchers)	12-oz. dinner	224
PEPPER, SWEET, raw:		
Green, whole	1 lb.	82
Red, whole	1 lb.	112
PERCH:		
Raw, whole:		
White	1 lb.	193
Yellow	1 lb.	161
Frozen, breaded (Gorton)	11-oz. pkg.	339
PERNOD (Julius Wile) 90 proof	1 fl. oz.	79
PERSIMMON, Japanese or Kaki:		
With seeds	1 lb.	286
Seedless	1 lb.	293

*Prepared as Package Directs

Food and Description	Measure or Quantity	Calories
PHEASANT, raw, ready-to-cook	1 lb.	596
PICKLE:		
Cucumber, fresh or bread & butter (Aunt Jane's)	4 slices or sticks	21
Dill, *L & S*	1 large pickle	15
Dill, candied (Smucker's)	4" pickle	46
Kosher dill (Smucker's)	3½" pickle	8
Sour (Heinz)	2" pickle	1
Sweet:		
Gherkin (Bond's)	1 pickle	19
Mixed (Heinz)	3 pieces	23
PIECRUST:		
(Mrs. Smith's)	8" shell	692
(Mrs. Smith's) old fashioned	9" shell	867
(Mrs. Smith's)	10" shell	1177
PIECRUST MIX:		
*Graham cracker (Betty Crocker)	1 crust	954
*(Flako)	9" shell	726
PIGS FEET, pickled (Hormel)	1-pt. can	442
PIKE, raw:		
Blue, whole	1 lb.	180
Northern, whole	1 lb.	104
Walleye, whole	1 lb.	240
PILLSBURY INSTANT BREAKFAST	1 oz.	101
PIMIENTO (Ortega)	¼ cup	6
PINA COLADA mix (Party Tyme)	½-oz. pkg.	50
PINCH of HERBS (Lawry's)	2.2-oz. pkg.	212
PINEAPPLE:		
Fresh, whole	1 lb.	123
Canned:		
Juice pack:		
Chunks or crushed (Dole)	½ cup (includes 2½ T. juice)	66

*Prepared as Package Directs

Food and Description	Measure or Quantity	Calories
Slices (Dole)	2 med. slices & 2½ T. juice	84
Heavy syrup (Del Monte)	½ cup	100
Canned, unsweetened (S and W) *Nutradiet*	2½ slices	56
PINEAPPLE, CANDIED (Liberty)	1 oz.	93
PINEAPPLE & GRAPEFRUIT JUICE DRINK (Dole) regular or pink	6-fl.-oz. can	100
PINEAPPLE JUICE:		
(Heinz)	5½-fl.-oz. can	101
(Dole)	6-fl.-oz. can	103
PINEAPPLE PIE (Morton)	46-oz. pie	3192
PINEAPPLE PIE FILLING:		
(Comstock)	½ cup	140
(Lucky Leaf)	8 oz.	240
PINE NUT		
Pignolias, shelled	¼ lb.	626
Piñon, shelled	¼ lb.	720
PISTACHIO NUT:		
In shell	¼ lb.	337
Dry, roasted (Flavor House)	1 oz.	168
PIZZA PIE, frozen:		
With cheese (Chef Boy-Ar-Dee)	12½" pie	786
With cheese (Kraft)	14-oz. pie	826
With pepperoni (Chef Boy-Ar-Dee)	14-oz. pie	900
With sausage, *Pee Wee* (Kraft)	2½-oz. pie	191
PIZZA PIE MIX:		
*With cheese (Chef Boy-Ar-Dee)	15½-oz. pie	935
*With sausage (Chef Boy-Ar-Dee)	17-oz. pie	1110

*Prepared as Package Directs

Food and Description	Measure or Quantity	Calories
PIZZA SAUCE:		
(Chef Boy-Ar-Dee)	10½-oz. can	232
Mix (French's)	1-oz. pkg.	77
PIZZARIA MIX (Hunt's) *Skillet*	14.1-oz. pkg.	507
PLANTAIN, whole	1 lb.	389
PLUM:		
Fresh, Japanese & hybrid	1 lb.	205
Fresh, prune-type	1 lb.	320
Canned, heavy syrup (Del Monte)	½ cup	112
Canned, unsweetened (Tillie Lewis)	½ cup	63
PLUM PUDDING (Crosse & Blackwell)	4 oz.	340
POLISH-STYLE SAUSAGE:		
(Oscar Mayer) all meat	1 oz.	81
Kolbase (Hormel)	1 oz.	80
POLYNESIAN-STYLE DINNER (Swanson)	11¾-oz. dinner	512
POMEGRANATE, whole	1 lb.	160
POMMARD WINE:		
(B & G) 13% alcohol	3 fl. oz.	67
(Chanson) 11½% alcohol	3 fl. oz.	60
POMPANO, raw, whole	1 lb.	422
POPCORN:		
(Jiffy Pop)	5-oz. pkg.	488
(Tom Houston)	1 cup	68
Buttered (Jiffy Pop)	5-oz. pkg.	494
Cracker Jack	1 cup	57
Cheese (Wise)	⅝-oz. bag	90
*POPOVER, mix (Flako)	1 pkg.	966
PORGY, whole	1 lb.	208

*Prepared as Package Directs

Food and Description	Measure or Quantity	Calories
PORK:		
Fresh, raw:		
Boston butt	1 lb.	1220
Ham, raw	1 lb.	1188
Loin, raw	1 lb.	1065
Picnic, raw	1 lb.	1083
Spareribs, raw with bone	1 lb.	976
Cured:		
Boston butt, raw	1 lb.	1227
Ham:		
Raw	1 lb.	1100
Fully cooked, bone-in (Hormel)	1 lb.	828
Fully cooked, boneless:		
Parti-Style (Armour Star)	1 lb.	668
Festival, smoked (Wilson)	1 lb.	764
Picnic:		
Raw	1 lb.	1060
Canned (Hormel)	3-lb. can	2472
PORK DINNER (Swanson)	10-oz. dinner	460
PORK RINDS, *Baken·ets*	1 oz.	147
PORK SAUSAGE:		
(Armour Star)	1-oz. sausage	133
Little Friers (Oscar Mayer)	1-oz. link	129
PORK, SWEET & SOUR (Chun King)	15-oz. pkg.	440
PORT WINE:		
(Gallo) 16% alcohol	3 fl. oz.	94
(Italian Swiss Colony-Gold Medal) 19.7% alcohol	3 fl. oz.	130
(Louis M. Martini) 19½% alcohol	3 fl. oz.	165
(Robertson's) tawny, 21% alcohol	3 fl. oz.	145
POST TOASTIES (Post)	1 oz.	108
***POSTUM**	1 cup	16

*Prepared as Package Directs

Food and Description	Measure or Quantity	Calories
POTATO:		
Raw, whole	1 lb.	279
Canned, white (Butter Kernel)	3-4 small potatoes	96
Frozen:		
Au gratin (Stouffer's)	11½-oz. pkg.	304
Stuffed, baked, with cheese or sour cream (Holloway House)	1 potato	296
Stuffed, baked, with sour cream & chives (Holloway House)	1 potato	296
POTATO CHIP:		
(Pringle's)	10 chips	73
(Wise)	1-oz. bag	156
Barbecue (Wise)	1-oz. bag	152
Ridgies (Wise)	1 oz. bag	155
POTATO MIX:		
Au gratin (French's)	5½-oz. pkg.	573
Mashed, country-style (French's)	2⅔ -oz. pkg.	267
Scalloped (French's)	5⅝-oz. pkg.	552
Whipped (Borden)	1 cup	208
POTATO PANCAKE MIX (French's)	3-oz. pkg.	284
POTATO SALAD, canned (Nalley's)	4 oz.	178
POTATO STICK:		
(Durkee) *O & C*	1⅝-oz. can	253
Julienne (Wise)	1-oz. bag	151
POUILLY-FUISSE WINE (B & G) 12½% alcohol	3 fl. oz.	64
POUILLY-FUME (B & G) 12% alcohol	3 fl. oz.	60
POUND CAKE:		
Plain (Drake's)	9-oz. cake	910
Plain (Sara Lee)	1 oz.	110
PRESERVE (Kraft)	1 oz.	78

*Prepared as Package Directs

Food and Description	Measure or Quantity	Calories
PRETZEL:		
(Nabisco) *Mister Salty*, Dutch	½-oz. piece	51
(Nabisco) *Mister Salty Veri-Thin*, sticks	1 piece	1
(Old London) nuggets	2-oz. bag	211
PRODUCT 19 (Kellogg's)	1 oz.	105
·PRUNE:		
Dried (Del Monte)	½ cup	236
Canned (Sunsweet)	1 cup	300
PRUNE JUICE:		
(Bennett's)	½ cup	99
(Heinz)	5½-fl.-oz. can	119
PULIGNY MONTRACHET WINE		
(B & G) 12% alcohol	3 fl. oz.	61
PUMPKIN:		
Fresh, whole	1 lb.	83
Canned (Libby's)	½ cup	41
PUMPKIN PIE:		
(Banquet)	5-oz. serving	306
(Morton)	20-oz. pie	1002
(Mrs. Smith's)	8″ pie	1453
PUMPKIN PIE FILLING		
(Comstock)	1 cup	366
PUMPKIN SEED, hulled	¼ lb.	627

Q

QUAKE, cereal	1 oz.	119
QUININE SOFT DRINK or TONIC WATER:		
Sweetened:		
(Canada Dry)	6 fl. oz.	68
(Dr. Brown's) (Hoffman) (Schweppes)	6 fl. oz.	66

*Prepared as Package Directs

Food and Description	Measure or Quantity	Calories
(Fanta)	6 fl. oz.	62
(Kirsch)	6 fl. oz.	71
(Shasta)	6 fl. oz.	57
(Yukon Club)	6 fl. oz.	67
Low calorie (No-Cal)	6 fl. oz.	2

R

RABBIT, ready-to-cook	1 lb.	581
RADISH, without tops	½ lb.	34
RAISIN:		
Seeded, Muscat (Sun-Maid)	15-oz. pkg.	1140
Seedless, golden (Sun-Maid)	15-oz. pkg.	1248
RASPBERRY:		
Fresh, black	½ lb.	160
Fresh, red	½ lb.	126
Frozen (Birds Eye)	½ cup	148
RASPBERRY SOFT DRINK:		
Sweetened:		
(Clicquot Club) (Cott) (Mission)	6 fl. oz.	98
(Dr. Brown's)	6 fl. oz.	86
(Hoffman) (Shasta) (Yukon Club)	6 fl. oz.	89
(Kirsch)	6 fl. oz.	88
Low calorie:		
(Clicquot Club) (Cott) (Mission) (No-Cal)	6 fl. oz.	3
(Dr. Brown's) (Hoffman) (Key Food) (Waldbaum)	6 fl. oz.	2
(Shasta)	6 fl. oz.	<1
RASPBERRY TURNOVER		
(Pepperidge Farm)	1 turnover	369
RAVIOLI:		
Meat (Chef Boy-Ar-Dee)	40-oz. can	1055
Cheese (Chef Boy-Ar-Dee)	15-oz. can	524
Frozen:		
Beef (Kraft)	12½-oz. pkg.	411
Cheese (Kraft)	12½-oz. pkg.	407

*Prepared as Package Directs

Food and Description	Measure or Quantity	Calories
RED & GRAY SNAPPER, whole	1 lb.	219
RELISH:		
Barbecue (Heinz)	1 T.	35
Corn (Crosse & Blackwell)	1 T.	15
Hamburger (Del Monte)	1 T.	33
Hot dog (Heinz)	1 T.	17
India (Crosse & Blackwell)	1 T.	26
Piccalilli (Heinz)	1 T.	23
Sweet (Lutz & Schramm)	1 T.	14
RHINE WINE:		
(Gallo) Rhine Garten, 12% alcohol	3 fl. oz.	59
(Italian Swiss Colony-Gold Medal)		
11.6% alcohol	3 fl. oz.	59
(Taylor) 12½% alcohol	3 fl. oz.	69
RHUBARB:		
Fresh, partly trimmed	1 lb.	54
Frozen (Birds Eye)	½ cup	84
RICE:		
Brown, raw	1 oz.	102
White, raw:		
Instant	1 oz.	106
Parboiled, long-grain	1 oz.	105
Regular	1 oz.	102
White & wild (Green Giant)	12-oz. pkg.	321
RICE CHEX (Ralston)	1 oz.	107
RICE, FRIED:		
Frozen:		
With almonds (Green Giant)	12-oz. pkg.	492
With chicken (Chun King)	10-oz. pkg.	618
With meat (Chun King)	10-oz. pkg.	634
With shrimp (Temple)	1 cup	297
Seasoning mix (Durkee)	1-oz. pkg.	62
RICE KRISPIES (Kellogg's)	1 oz.	109

*Prepared as Package Directs

Food and Description	Measure or Quantity	Calories
*RICE MIX, SPANISH (Uncle Ben's) with added butter	½ cup	129
RICE & PEAS with MUSH- ROOMS (Green Giant)	12-oz. pkg.	354
RICE PILAF (Green Giant)	12-oz. pkg.	348
RICE, PUFFED (Checker) (Sunland) (Whiffs)	1 oz.	112
RICE PUDDING (Hunt's)	5-oz. can	240
RICE, SPANISH:		
(Heinz)	8¾-oz. can	196
Frozen (Green Giant)	12-oz. pkg.	261
Seasoning mix (Lawry's)	1½-oz. pkg.	125
RICE VERDI (Green Giant)	12-oz. pkg.	402
RIESLING WINE (Wilm) 11-14% alcohol	3 fl. oz.	66
RING DINGS (Drake's)	2¾-oz. cake	350
RIPPLE WINE, red (Gallo)	3 fl. oz.	56
ROAST 'n BOAST (General Foods):		
For beef	1½-oz. pkg.	129
For chicken	1⅜-oz. pkg.	119
For pork	1¾-oz. pkg.	145
For stew	1½-oz. pkg.	126
ROCKFISH, raw, meat only	1 lb.	440
ROE, cod or shad, raw	4 oz.	147
ROLAIDS (Warner-Lambert)	1 piece	4
ROLL & BUN:		
Barbeque (Arnold)	1 bun	132
Brown & serve (Wonder)	1 roll	79

*Prepared as Package Directs

Food and Description	Measure or Quantity	Calories
Butter crescent (Pepperidge Farm)	1 roll	127
Butterfly (Pepperidge Farm)	1 roll	58
Cinnamon, iced (Van de Kamp's)	1 roll	127
Cinnamon nut (Pepperidge Farm)	1 bun	92
Club (Pepperidge Farm)	1 roll	114
Deli Twist (Arnold)	1 roll	115
Diet Size (Arnold)	1 roll	40
Dinner (Arnold)	1 roll	71
Dinner (Pepperidge Farm)	1 roll	61
Dutch Egg, sandwich (Arnold)	1 bun	143
Finger:		
(Arnold) handipan	1 roll	61
Egg (Arnold) family	1 roll	62
(Sara Lee)	1 oz.	84
Frankfurter:		
(Arnold)	1 roll	121
New England (Arnold)	1 roll	130
(Pepperidge Farm)	1 roll	117
(Wonder)	1 bun	122
French:		
Butter (Van de Kamp's)	1 roll	105
Triple (Pepperidge Farm)	1 roll	253
Twin (Pepperidge Farm)	1 roll	363
Golden Twist (Pepperidge Farm)	1 roll	127
Hamburger:		
(Pepperidge Farm)	1 roll	112
(Wonder)	1 bun	122
Hard (Levy's)	1 roll	130
Hearth (Pepperidge Farm)	1 roll	59
Honey, frozen (Morton)	1 serving	170
Hot Cross (Van de Kamp's)	1 bun	63
Kaiser, brown & serve (Arnold)	1 roll	132
Old Fashioned (Pepperidge Farm)	1 roll	36
Parker (Arnold) handipan	1 roll	63
Parkerhouse (Sara Lee)	1 oz.	83
Party Pan (Pepperidge Farm):		
Plain	1 roll	34
Poppy	1 roll	34
Pecan, coffee (Pepperidge Farm)	1 bun	195
Sandwich, soft (Arnold)	1 roll	135
Sesame crisp (Pepperidge Farm):		
Mid-west	1 roll	74

*Prepared as Package Directs

Food and Description	Measure or Quantity	Calories
East	1 roll	71
Sesame seed (Sara Lee)	1 oz.	84
Soft (Arnold) handipan	1 roll	58
Sourdough, French (Van de Kamp's)	1 roll	130

ROLL DOUGH, refrigerated:
Cinnamon with icing (Pillsbury)	1 oz.	100
Dinner (Pillsbury):		
Buttermilk	1 oz.	80
Crescent	1 oz.	94
Parkerhouse	1 oz.	76
Snowflake	1 oz.	84

ROLL MIX (Pillsbury) hot	1 oz.	113

ROOT BEER SOFT DRINK:
Sweetened:		
(Canada Dry) *Rooti*	6 fl. oz.	76
(Clicquot Club) (Cott) (Mission)	6 fl. oz.	85
(Dad's)	6 fl. oz.	79
(Dr. Brown's) (Fanta) (Hoffman) (Key Food) (Nedick's) (Waldbaum)	6 fl. oz.	77
(Hires)	6 fl. oz.	75
(Kirsch)	6 fl. oz.	71
(Nehi)	6 fl. oz.	95
(Salute)	6 fl. oz.	90
(Shasta) draft	6 fl. oz.	84
(Yukon Club)	6 fl. oz.	81
Low calorie:		
(Canada Dry) (Clicquot Club) (Cott) (Dad's) (Hoffman) (Mission) (No-Cal) (Shasta) (Yukon Club)	6 fl. oz.	<1

ROSE WINE:
(Antinori) 12% alcohol	3 fl. oz.	84
(Gallo) 13% alcohol	3 fl. oz.	55
(Great Western) 12.5% alcohol	3 fl. oz.	88
(Mogen David) 12% alcohol	3 fl. oz.	75
(Taylor) 12½% alcohol	3 fl. oz.	69

*Prepared as Package Directs

Food and Description	Measure or Quantity	Calories
RUSK (Nabisco)	1 piece	49
RUTABAGA, raw, without tops	1 lb.	177

S

Food and Description	Measure or Quantity	Calories
SABLEFISH, whole	1 lb.	362
SAINT-EMILION WINE (B & G) 12% alcohol	3 fl. oz.	63
SALAD DRESSING:		
(Bennett's)	1 T.	51
Blendaise (Marzetti)	1 T.	60
Bleu or blue cheese:		
(Kraft) Imperial	1 T.	68
(Lawry's)	1 T.	57
Caesar (Kraft)	1 T.	63
Caesar (Lawry's)	1 T.	70
Coleslaw (Kraft)	1 T.	62
French:		
(Best Foods) (Hellmann's)	1 T.	65
(Wish-Bone) deluxe	1 T.	59
(Wish-Bone) garlic	1 T.	88
Garlic, French (Hellmann's)	1 T.	68
Green Goddess:		
(Kraft)	1 T.	75
(Wish-Bone)	1 T.	68
Italian:		
(Lawry's)	1 T.	80
(Lawry's) with cheese	1 T.	60
(Wish-Bone)	1 T.	75
Mayonnaise, imitation (Healthlife)	.5 oz.	61
Miracle Whip (Kraft)	1 T.	69
Oil & vinegar (Kraft)	1 T.	65
Roquefort (Marzetti)	1 T.	80
Russian (Kraft) creamy	1 T.	68
(Saffola)	1 T.	52
Thousand Island:		
(Best Foods)	1 T.	60
(Lawry's)	1 T.	69

*Prepared as Package Directs

Food and Description	Measure or Quantity	Calories
SALAD DRESSING, DIETETIC		
or LOW CALORIE:		
Bleu or blue:		
(Frenchette) chunky	1 T.	22
(Kraft)	1 T.	13
(Slim-ette)	1 T.	12
Caesar (Frenchette)	1 T.	33
Chef style (Kraft)	1 T.	16
Chef's (Tillie Lewis)	1 T.	2
Diet Mayo 7 (Bennett's)	1 T.	23
French:		
(Bennett's)	1 T.	21
(Frenchette)	1 T.	10
Green Goddess (Slim-ette)	1 T.	12
Italian:		
Italianette (Frenchette)	1 T.	7
(Tillie Lewis)	1 T.	1
(Wish-Bone)	1 T.	16
Mayonette Gold (Frenchette)	1 T.	33
Thousand Island:		
(Frenchette)	1 T.	22
(Kraft)	1 T.	28
SALAD SEASONING (Durkee)	1 tsp.	4
SALAMI:		
Cotto, all meat (Oscar Mayer)	.8-oz. slice	55
Dilusso Genoa (Hormel)	1 oz.	120
Machiaeh brand, pure beef		
(Oscar Mayer)	.8-oz. slice	60
SALISBURY STEAK:		
(Banquet)	2-lb. pkg.	1524
(Holloway House)	7-oz. steak	320
(Swanson) *Hungry Man*	17-oz. dinner	943
(Morton) 3-course	1-lb. 1-oz. dinner	612
SALMON:		
Chinook or King, steak, raw	1 lb.	886
Chinook or King, canned	4 oz.	238
Chum, canned	4 oz.	158
Coho, canned (Icy Point)	3¾-oz. can	162

*Prepared as Package Directs

Pink or Humpback:		
Raw, steak	1 lb.	475
Canned, (Del Monte)	7¾-oz. can	268
Canned (Icy Point) (Pink Beauty)	7¾-oz. can	310
Sockeye or Red or Blueback canned:		
(Del Monte)	7¾-oz. can	304
(Icy Point) (Pillar Rock)	7¾-oz. can	376
SALMON, SMOKED:		
Lox, drained (Vita)	4-oz. jar	136
Nova, drained (Vita)	4-oz. can	221
SALT:		
Butter flavored (Durkee)	1 tsp.	3
Garlic (Lawry's)	2.9-oz. pkg.	116
Onion (Lawry's)	3-oz. pkg.	106
Seasoned (Lawry's)	3-oz. pkg.	21
SALT PORK	1 lb.	3410
SANDWICH SPREAD:		
(Kraft)	1 oz.	105
(Nalley's)	1 oz.	100
Corned beef (Carnation)	7½-oz. can	480
Ham salad (Carnation)	7½-oz. can	400
Tuna salad (Carnation)	7½-oz. can	450
SANGRIA MIX (Party Tyme)	½-oz. pkg.	53
SARDINE:		
Moroccan, skinless (Cresca):		
In olive oil	3¾-oz. can	341
In water	3¾-oz. can	165
Norwegian, canned:		
In mustard sauce (Underwood)	3¾-oz. can	196
In oil, drained (Underwood)	3¾-oz. can	232
In tomato sauce (Underwood)	3¾-oz. can	169
SAUCE:		
A1	1 T.	14
Barbecue:		
(French's) smoky	1 T.	15

*Prepared as Package Directs

Food and Description	Measure or Quantity	Calories
(General Foods) hickory smoke, *Open Pit*	1 T.	27
(Heinz) with onions, hickory smoke	1 T.	18
(Kraft) hickory smoke	1 T.	34
Escoffier Sauce Diable	1 T.	16
Escoffier Sauce Robert	1 T.	23
Famous (Durkee)	1 T.	72
57 (Heinz)	1 T.	14
H.P. Steak Sauce (Lea & Perrins)	1 T.	20
Marinara (Chef Boy-Ar-Dee)	15-oz. can	272
Seafood cocktail (Crosse & Blackwell)	1 T.	22
Sloppy Joe (Contadina)	1 T.	9
Soy (Chun King)	1 T.	6
Steak (Crosse & Blackwell)	1 T.	21
Sweet & sour (La Choy)	1 T.	30
Tartar (Best Foods) (Hellmann's)	1 T.	74
White, medium	1 cup	413
Worcestershire (Lea & Perrins)	1 T.	12

SAUCE MIX:

Food and Description	Measure or Quantity	Calories
*A la King (Durkee)	1.1-oz. pkg.	135
*Barbecue (Kraft)	1 oz.	32
Cheese (French's)	1¼-oz. pkg.	165
Hollandaise (French's)	1⅛-oz. pkg.	192
*Mushroom (Betty Crocker)	1 cup	144
*Sour Cream (Kraft)	1 oz.	61
Stroganoff (French's)	1¾-oz. pkg.	192
*Sweet-sour (Durkee)	2-oz. pkg.	230
*White (Durkee)	1½-oz. pkg.	381

SAUERKRAUT (Stokely-Van Camp) 1 cup 40

SAUSAGE:

Food and Description	Measure or Quantity	Calories
Breakfast (Hormel)	8-oz. can	838
Brown 'n serve (Hormel)	1 piece	78
In sauce, canned (Prince)	3.7-oz. can	187

SAUTERNES:

Food and Description	Measure or Quantity	Calories
(B & G) 13% alcohol	3 fl. oz.	95
(Gallo) haut, 12% alcohol	3 fl. oz.	67
(Taylor) 12½% alcohol	3 fl. oz.	81

*Prepared as Package Directs

SCALLOP:
Raw, muscle only	1 lb.	368
Frozen:		
Breaded, fried (Mrs. Paul's)	7-oz. pkg.	412
Crisps (Gorton)	7-oz. pkg.	310

SCOTCH SOUR COCKTAIL:
(National Distillers) *Duet*, 12½% alcohol	8-fl.-oz. can	272
(Party Tyme) 12½% alcohol	2 fl. oz.	65

SCRAPPLE (Oscar Mayer)   4 oz.   202

SCREWDRIVER:
(National Distillers) *Duet*, 12½% alcohol	8-fl.-oz. can	288
(Party Tyme) 12½% alcohol	2 fl. oz.	69
Mix (Bar-Tender's)	1 serving	70

SEABASS, WHITE, raw, meat only   1 lb.   436

SEAFOOD PLATTER, fried (Mrs. Paul's)   9-oz. pkg.   517

SENEGALESE SOUP (Crosse & Blackwell)   13-oz. can   122

SESAME SEED, hulled   1 oz.   165

SEVEN-UP:
Regular	6 fl. oz.	73
Low calorie	6 fl. oz.	21

SHAD, whole   1 lb.   370

SHAKE 'N BAKE:
Chicken-coating	2⅜-oz. pkg.	276
Fish-coating	2-oz. pkg.	224
Hamburger-coating	2-oz. pkg.	158
Pork-coating	2⅜-oz. pkg.	260

*Prepared as Package Directs

Food and Description	Measure or Quantity	Calories
SHALLOT, raw, whole	¼ lb.	72
SHERBET (Borden) (Meadow Gold) (Sealtest)	1 pint	480
SHERRY:		
Cocktail (Gold Seal) 19% alcohol	3 fl. oz.	122
Cream:		
(Gallo) 20% alcohol	3 fl. oz.	111
(Great Western) Solera, 18% alcohol	3 fl. oz.	138
(Taylor) 19½% alcohol	3 fl. oz.	150
Dry:		
(Italian Swiss Colony-Gold Medal) 19.7% alcohol	3 fl. oz.	104
(Williams & Humbert) 20½% alcohol	3 fl. oz.	120
Dry Sack (Williams & Humbert) 20½% alcohol	3 fl. oz.	120
Medium:		
(Italian Swiss Colony-Private Label) 19.8% alcohol	3 fl. oz.	108
(Taylor) 19½% alcohol	3 fl. oz.	132
SHREDDED WHEAT:		
(Kellogg's) *Mini-Wheats*	1 oz.	108
(Nabisco)	1 biscuit	86
(Nabisco) *Spoon Size*	1 oz.	107
(Quaker)	2 biscuits	135
SHRIMP:		
Raw, whole	1 lb.	285
Cocktail, tiny, drained (Icy Point) (Pillar Rock) (Snow Mist)	4½-oz. can	148
Frozen:		
Breaded (Gorton)	1-lb. pkg.	632
Fried (Mrs. Paul's)	4 oz.	258
Scampi (Gorton)	7½-oz. pkg.	570
SHRIMP CAKE (Mrs. Paul's)	10-oz. pkg.	630

*Prepared as Package Directs

Food and Description	Measure or Quantity	Calories
SHRIMP COCKTAIL:		
(Sau-Sea)	4-oz. jar	107
(Sea Snack)	4-oz. jar	110
SHRIMP DINNER:		
(Morton)	7¾-oz. dinner	379
(Swanson)	8-oz. dinner	358
SHRIMP PASTE	1 oz.	51
SHRIMP PUFF (Durkee)	1 piece	44
SLENDER (Carnation):		
Dry	1 pkg.	104
Liquid	10-fl.-oz. can	225
SLIM JIM:		
Sausage	1 piece	83
Polish sausage, all beef	1 piece	108
SLOPPY JOE:		
(French's)	1½-oz. pkg.	117
(Lawry's)	1½-oz. pkg.	139
(McCormick)	1⁵/₁₆-oz. pkg.	112
SMELT, raw, whole	1 lb.	244
SMOKIE SAUSAGE:		
(Oscar Mayer):		
8 links per ¾ lb.	1 link	131
7 links per 5 oz.	1 link	61
(Wilson)	1 oz.	84
SNO BALL (Hostess)	1 cake	135
SOAVE WINE (Antinori) 12% alcohol	3 fl. oz.	84
SOFT SWIRL (Jell-O):		
*All flavors except chocolate	½ cup	168
*Chocolate	½ cup	190

*Prepared as Package Directs

Food and Description	Measure or Quantity	Calories
SOLE:		
Raw, whole	1 lb.	118
Raw, meat only	1 lb.	360
Frozen:		
(Gorton)	1-lb. pkg.	360
(Weight Watchers)	18-oz. dinner	279
In lemon butter (Gorton)	9-oz. pkg.	441
SOUP BASE (Wyler's) beef & chicken	1 tsp.	29
SOUTHERN COMFORT:		
86 proof	1 fl. oz.	84
100 proof	1 fl. oz.	96
SOYBEAN:		
Young seeds, raw	1 lb.	322
Mature seeds, raw	1 lb.	1828
Roasted, *Soy Town*	1 oz.	152
SPAGHETTI, dry	1 oz.	105
SPAGHETTI DINNER:		
*With meat balls (Chef Boy-Ar-Dee)	8¾-oz. pkg.	362
*With meat sauce (Kraft) *Deluxe*	8 oz.	302
Frozen, with meat balls:		
(Banquet)	11.5-oz. dinner	423
(Morton)	11-oz. dinner	368
(Swanson)	12-oz. dinner	323
SPAGHETTI & FRANKFURTERS (Heinz)	8½-oz. can	308
SPAGHETTI & GROUND BEEF (Chef Boy-Ar-Dee)	15-oz. can	384
SPAGHETTI & MEATBALLS:		
Canned:		
(Austex)	15½-oz. can	437
(Franco-American)	1 cup	264
SpaghettiO's (Franco-American)	1 cup	215
Frozen (Buitoni)	8 oz.	262

*Prepared as Package Directs

Food and Description	Measure or Quantity	Calories
SPAGHETTI with MEAT SAUCE:		
Canned (Heinz)	8½-oz. can	207
Frozen:		
(Banquet)	2-lb. pkg.	1324
(Kraft)	12½-oz. pkg.	343
(Morton)	20-oz. casserole	722
*SPAGHETTI MIX (Kraft)	4 oz.	121
SPAGHETTI SAUCE:		
Clam, red (Buitoni)	4 oz.	106
Clam, white (Buitoni)	4 oz.	140
Italian (Contadina)	4 fl. oz.	76
Meat:		
(Chef Boy-Ar-Dee)	15-oz. can	372
(Prince)	1 cup	288
Meatball (Chef Boy-Ar-Dee)	15-oz. can	606
Meatless or plain:		
(Heinz)	1 cup	196
(Ronzoni)	8 oz.	220
Mushroom (Chef Boy-Ar-Dee)	15-oz. can	272
SPAGHETTI SAUCE MIX:		
(McCormick)	1½-oz. pkg.	147
Italian (French's)	1½-oz. pkg.	108
*Prepared without oil (Spatini)	1 cup	100
*Prepared with oil (Spatini)	1 cup	152
With mushrooms (Lawry's)	1½-oz. pkg.	147
SPAGHETTI SAUCE WITH TOMATO:		
(Van Camp)	1 cup	168
With cheese (Chef Boy-Ar-Dee)	40-oz. can	80
SPAM:		
Regular	3 oz.	260
Spread	1 oz.	80
SPANISH-STYLE VEGETABLES		
(Birds Eye)	10-oz. pkg.	255
SPECIAL K (Kellogg's)	1 oz.	109

*Prepared as Package Directs

Food and Description	Measure or Quantity	Calories
*SPICE CAKE MIX (Duncan Hines)	1 cake	2388
SPINACH:		
Raw, packaged	1 lb.	118
Canned (Stokely-Van Camp)	1 cup	42
Frozen:		
(Birds Eye)	10-oz. pkg.	69
In cream sauce (Green Giant)	10-oz. pkg.	171
Leaf (Birds Eye)	10-oz. pkg.	69
Leaf, creamed (Birds Eye)	9-oz. pkg.	183
Leaf, in butter sauce (Green Giant)	10-oz. pkg.	117
SPINACH SOUFFLE (Stouffer's)	12-oz. pkg.	484
SPOT, fillets	1 lb.	993
SPRITE, soft drink	6 fl. oz.	70
SQUAB, dressed	1 lb.	569
SQUASH, SUMMER:		
Fresh, crookneck & straightneck	1 lb.	89
Fresh, scallop	1 lb.	93
Fresh, zucchini & cocozelle	1 lb.	73
Canned, zucchini in tomato sauce (Del Monte)	1 cup	50
Frozen:		
Parmesan, zucchini (Mrs. Paul's)	12-oz. pkg.	259
Summer squash (Birds Eye)	10-oz. pkg.	60
SQUASH, WINTER:		
Acorn	1 lb.	152
Butternut	1 lb.	171
Hubbard	1 lb.	117
Frozen (Birds Eye)	12-oz. pkg.	129
START	½ cup	60
STRAWBERRY:		
Fresh, whole	1 lb.	161

*Prepared as Package Directs

Food and Description	Measure or Quantity	Calories
Frozen:		
Whole (Birds Eye)	1-lb. pkg.	404
Halves (Birds Eye)	1-lb. pkg.	486
STRAWBERRY ICE CREAM:		
(Meadow Gold) 10% fat	1 pt.	504
(Sealtest)	1 pt.	532
STRAWBERRY PIE:		
(Morton)	20-oz. pie	1518
Cream (Morton)	14.4-oz. pie	988
STRAWBERRY PIE FILLING:		
(Comstock)	1 cup	318
(Lucky Leaf)	8 oz.	248
STRAWBERRY-RHUBARB PIE:		
(Morton)	46-oz. pie	3464
(Mrs. Smith's)	10″ pie	3354
STRAWBERRY-RHUBARB PIE FILLING (Lucky Leaf)	8 oz.	258
STRAWBERRY SOFT DRINK:*		
Sweetened:		
(Canada Dry) (Fanta)	6 fl. oz.	88
(Clicquot Club) (Cott) (Mission)	6 fl. oz.	98
(Hoffman)	6 fl. oz.	89
(Shasta)	6 fl. oz.	80
(Yoo-Hoo)	6 fl. oz.	90
High-protein (Yoo-Hoo)	6 fl. oz.	114
(Yukon Club)	6 fl. oz.	92
Low calorie:		
(Canada Dry) (Hoffman) (Shasta)	6 fl. oz.	<1
(Clicquot Club) (Cott) (Mission)	6 fl. oz.	3
STRAWBERRY TURNOVER		
(Pepperidge Farm)	1 turnover	326
STRUDEL, frozen (Pepperidge Farm):		
Apple	1 strudel	1212

*Prepared as Package Directs

Food and Description	Measure or Quantity	Calories
Blueberry	1 strudel	1440
Cherry	1 strudel	1224
Pineapple-cheese	1 strudel	1254
STURGEON:		
Section	1 lb.	362
Smoked	1 lb	676
SUCCOTASH, frozen (Birds Eye)	10-oz. pkg.	261
SUGAR:		
Brown	1 lb.	1692
Confectioners' or granulated	1 lb.	1746
Maple	1 lb.	1579
SUGAR CHEX, cereal	1 oz.	119
SUGAR FROSTED FLAKES (Kellogg's)	1 oz.	109
SUGAR JETS (General Mills)	1 oz.	111
SUGAR POPS (Kellogg's)	1 oz.	112
SUGAR SMACKS (Kellogg's)	1 oz.	112
SUGAR SPARKLED TWINKLES (General Mills)	1 oz.	112
SUGAR SUBSTITUTE:		
(Adolph's); *Sweetnin'* (Tillie Lewis)	1 tsp.	0
Superose (Whitlock); (Weight Watchers)	1 packet	4
SUNFLOWER SEED:		
In hulls	¼ lb.	343
Hulled	1 oz.	159
SWEETBREADS:		
Beef	1 lb.	939
Calf	1 lb.	426
Lamb	1 lb.	426

*Prepared as Package Directs

SWEET POTATO:

Raw, unpared	1 lb.	419
Canned:		
Heavy syrup (Del Monte)	½ cup	138
Vacuum pack (Taylor's)	½ cup	135
Frozen:		
Candied (Mrs. Paul's)	12-oz. pkg.	417
Candied yams (Birds Eye)	12-oz. pkg.	645
With brown sugar glaze (Birds Eye)	10-oz. pkg.	435

SWISS STEAK, frozen:

(Stouffer's)	10-oz. pkg.	569
Dinner (Swanson)	10-oz. dinner	361

SWORDFISH, raw, meat only	1 lb.	535

T

TABASCO	¼ tsp.	<1
TACO, beef, frozen (Patio)	13½-oz. pkg.	1074
TACO FILLING (Gebhardt)	4 oz.	252

TACO SEASONING MIX:

(French's)	1¾-oz. pkg.	123
(Lawry's)	1¼-oz. pkg.	120

TAMALE:

(Armour Star)	15½-oz. can	620
(Wilson)	15½-oz. can	601
Frozen (Banquet) buffet	2-lb. pkg.	1488

***TANG,** orange	½ cup	61
TANGELO, juice from fruit	1 lb.	104
TANGERINE or MANDARIN ORANGE, fresh, whole	1 lb.	154
***TANGERINE JUICE** (Minute Maid) (Snow Crop)	½ cup	57

*Prepared as Package Directs

Food and Description	Measure or Quantity	Calories
TAPIOCA (Minute Tapioca)	1 T.	40
TAPIOCA PUDDING:		
Chilled (Sealtest)	4 oz.	130
Canned (Hunt's)	5-oz. can	166
*Mix, fluffy (Minute Tapioca)	½ cup	150
TEA:		
(Lipton)	1 bag	0
Instant:		
Nestea	1 tsp.	<1
*Lemon flavored (Lipton)	1 cup	3
TEAM	1 oz.	107
TEA MIX, iced:		
Nestea, any flavor	3 tsp.	58
*Lemon flavored (Lipton)	1 cup	102
THICK & FROSTY (General Foods)	1 cup	314
THUNDERBIRD WINE (Gallo):		
14% alcohol	3 fl. oz.	86
20% alcohol	3 fl. oz.	106
THURINGER, sausage, all meat		
(Oscar Mayer)	.8-oz. slice	74
TIA MARIA (Hiram Walker)		
63 proof	1 fl. oz.	92
TILEFISH, whole	1 lb.	183
TOASTER CAKE:		
Corn Treats (Arnold)	1.1-oz. piece	111
Toastee (Howard Johnson's):		
Blueberry	1 piece	121
Cinnamon raisin	1 piece	114
Corn	1 piece	112
Orange	1 piece	113
Pound	1 piece	111

*Prepared as Package Directs

Food and Description	Measure or Quantity	Calories
Toastette (Nabisco):		
Apple, blueberry, peach		
strawberry	1 piece	184
Brown sugar, cinnamon	1 piece	189
Cherry, orange marmalade	1 piece	182
Toast-r-Cake (Thomas):		
Bran	1 piece	116
Corn	1 piece	118
Orange	1 piece	117
TOASTERINO, frozen (Buitoni):		
Cheese, grilled	4 oz.	286
Pizzaburger	4 oz.	298
Sloppy Joe	4 oz.	295
TOMATO:		
Fresh, green	1 lb.	99
Fresh, ripe	1 lb.	100
Canned:		
Sliced (Contadina)	1 cup	72
Stewed (Del Monte)	1 cup	60
Whole (Stokely-Van Camp)	1 cup	46
TOMATO JUICE:		
(Heinz)	5½-fl.-oz. can	34
(Hunt's)	5½-fl.-oz. can	30
TOMATO JUICE COCKTAIL,		
Snap-E-Tom	6 fl. oz.	41
TOMATO PASTE (Contadina)	6-oz. can	144
TOMATO PUREE (Contadina)	1 cup	96
TOMATO SALAD, jellied		
(Contadina)	1 cup	120
TOMATO SAUCE:		
(Contadina)	1 cup	80
(Del Monte) plain	1 cup	60
(Del Monte) with mushrooms	1 cup	75
(Del Monte) with onions	1 cup	90

*Prepared as Package Directs

Food and Description	Measure or Quantity	Calories
(Del Monte) with tomato tidbits	1 cup	90
(Hunt's) plain	1 cup	78
(Hunt's) herb	1 cup	186
(Hunt's) special	1 cup	94
(Hunt's) with bits	1 cup	82
(Hunt's) with cheese	1 cup	107
(Hunt's) with mushrooms	1 cup	83
(Hunt's) with onions	1 cup	102

TOMATO SOUP:
(Campbell)	1 can	158
(Heinz) *Great American*	1 cup	168
Bisque (Campbell)	1 can	230

TOMATO SOUP MIX:
(Lipton) *Cup-a-Soup*	1 pkg.	79
*Vegetable, with noodles (Lipton)	1 cup	68

TOM COLLINS:
Mix (Party Tyme)	½-oz. pkg.	50
Soft drink (Canada Dry)	6 fl. oz.	61

TONGUE:
Beef, raw	1 lb.	714
Calf, raw	1 lb.	454
Lamb, raw	1 lb.	659

TONGUE, CANNED (Hormel)
TONGUE, CANNED (Hormel)	12-oz. can	802

TOPPING:
Butterscotch (Kraft)	1 oz.	84
Caramel (Kraft)	1 oz.	84
Chocolate fudge (Hershey's)	1 oz.	96
Marshmallow creme (Kraft)	1 oz.	90
Pecan in syrup (Smucker's)	1 T.	61
Pineapple (Kraft)	1 oz.	80
Walnut (Kraft)	1 oz.	113

TOPPING, WHIPPED:
(Birds Eye) *Cool Whip*	1 T.	16
(Lucky Whip)	1 T.	12

*Prepared as Package Directs

Food and Description	Measure or Quantity	Calories
TOPPING, WHIPPED, MIX:		
*(Dream Whip)	1 T.	14
*(Lucky Whip)	1 T.	10
TOTAL (General Mills)	1 oz.	100
TRIPE, beef, pickled	4 oz.	70
TRIPLE SEC LIQUEUR:		
(Bols) 78 proof	1 fl. oz.	101
(Garnier) 60 proof	1 fl. oz.	83
(Hiram Walker) 80 proof	1 fl. oz.	105
TRIX (General Mills)	1 oz.	110
TROUT:		
Raw, brook, whole	1 lb.	224
Frozen, boned	5-oz. trout	135
TUNA:		
Canned in oil:		
(Breast O' Chicken)	6½-oz. can	540
Chunk (Star-Kist)	6½-oz. can	535
Chunk, light (Chicken of the Sea)	6-oz. can	405
Canned in water:		
(Breast O' Chicken)	6½-oz. can	230
(Star-Kist)	6½-oz. can	207
TUNA CAKE (Mrs. Paul's)	10-oz. pkg.	689
TUNA PIE:		
(Banquet)	8-oz. pie	479
(Morton)	8-oz. pie	385
(Star-Kist)	8-oz. pie	450
TURBOT, GREENLAND:		
Raw, whole	1 lb.	344
(Weight Watchers)	18-oz. dinner	426
With apple (Weight Watchers)	9½-oz. luncheon	277

*Prepared as Package Directs

Food and Description	Measure or Quantity	Calories
TURKEY:		
Raw, ready-to-cook	1 lb.	722
Smoked, cooked, pressed (Oscar Mayer)	.8-oz. slice	23
Canned, boned (Swanson) with broth	5-oz. can	217
TURKEY DINNER, frozen:		
(Banquet)	11.5-oz. dinner	280
(Morton) 3-course	1-lb. 1-oz. dinner	634
(Swanson) 3-course	16-oz. dinner	501
(Weight Watchers)	18-oz. dinner	302
TURKEY FRICASSEE (Lynden Farms)	14.5-oz. can	366
TURKEY PIE, frozen:		
(Banquet)	2-lb. 4-oz. pie	1327
(Swanson) deep-dish	1-lb. pie	746
TURKEY TETRAZZINI (Stouffer's)	12-oz. pkg.	694
TURNIP, fresh, without tops	1 lb.	117
TURNIP GREENS, leaves & stems:		
Fresh	1 lb.	107
Frozen, chopped (Birds Eye)	10-oz. pkg.	66
TURTLE, GREEN, in shell	1 lb.	97
TWINKIE (Hostess) 12 to pkg.	1 cake	128

V

VALPOLICELLA WINE (Antinori)	3 fl. oz.	84
VANDERMINT (Park Avenue Imports) 60 proof	1 fl. oz.	90
VANILLA, pure extract (French's)	1 tsp.	13

*Prepared as Package Directs

Food and Description	Measure or Quantity	Calories
VANILLA ICE CREAM:		
(Borden) 10.5% fat	1 pt.	528
French (Prestige)	1 pt.	732
Fudge royale (Sealtest)	1 pt.	528
VANILLA ICE MILK (Borden)		
Lite-line	1 pt.	432
VANILLA PUDDING:		
Canned (Del Monte)	5-oz. can	190
Canned (Hunt's)	5-oz. can	238
Canned (My-T-Fine)	5-oz. can	192
*VANILLA PUDDING or PIE FILLING MIX (Royal)	½ cup	163
VEAL, raw, lean & fat:		
Chuck	1 lb. (weighed with bone)	628
Loin	1 lb. (weighed with bone)	681
Rib	1 lb. (weighed with bone)	723
Round & rump	1 lb. (weighed with bone)	573
VEAL DINNER:		
Parmigiana (Swanson)	12¼-oz. dinner	492
Breaded veal with spaghetti in tomato sauce (Swanson)	8¼-oz. pkg.	272
V-8 (Campbell)	¾ cup	31
VEGETABLES, MIXED:		
(Veg-All)	½ cup	39
Canned, Chinese, Chop Suey (Hung's)	4 oz.	20
Frozen:		
(Birds Eye)	10-oz. pkg.	150
In butter sauce (Green Giant)	10-oz. pkg.	180
Jubilee (Birds Eye)	10-oz. pkg.	414

*Prepared as Package Directs

Food and Description	Measure or Quantity	Calories
VEGETABLE SOUP:		
Canned, regular pack:		
*(Campbell) old fashioned	1 cup	70
*Beef (Heinz)	1 cup	66
With beef broth (Heinz) *Great*		
American	1 cup	144
Vegetarian:		
*(Campbell)	1 cup	71
*(Heinz)	1 cup	83
*Canned, dietetic pack (Slim-ette)	8 oz.	46
VENISON, raw	4 oz.	143
VERMOUTH:		
Dry & extra dry:		
(C & P) 19% alcohol	3 fl. oz.	90
(Lejon) 18.5% alcohol	3 fl. oz.	99
(Noilly Pratt) 19% alcohol	3 fl. oz.	101
Sweet:		
(C & P) 16% alcohol	3 fl. oz.	120
(Lejon) 18.5% alcohol	3 fl. oz.	134
(Noilly Pratt) 16% alcohol	3 fl. oz.	128
VERNORS, soft drink:		
Regular	6 fl. oz.	70
Low calorie	6 fl. oz.	1
VICHYSSOISE SOUP (Crosse & Blackwell)	13-oz. can	188
VIENNA SAUSAGE:		
(Armour Star)	5-oz. can	393
(Van Camp)	1 oz.	68
VINEGAR:		
Cider	½ cup	17
Distilled	½ cup	14
VODKA SCREWDRIVER (Old Mr. Boston) 25 proof	3 fl. oz.	117

*Prepared as Package Directs

Food and Description	Measure or Quantity	Calories

W

Food and Description	Measure or Quantity	Calories
WAFFLE, frozen, original (Aunt Jemima)	2 sections	117
WALNUT, English or Persian:		
In shell	1 lb.	1329
Shelled	4 oz.	738
(Diamond)	3-oz.	564
WATER CHESTNUT, CHINESE, raw	1 lb.	272
WATERCRESS, raw, whole	½ lb.	40
WATERMELON, fresh, whole	1 lb.	54
WATERMELON RIND (Crosse & Blackwell)	1 T.	38
WELSH RAREBIT, canned (Snow)	4 oz.	171
WHEATENA	½ cup	88
WHEAT GERM, cereal (Kretschmer)	1 oz.	106
WHEATIES (General Mills)	1 oz.	101
WHEAT, PUFFED, cereal (Quaker)	1 oz.	102
WHIP 'n CHILL (Jell-O):		
All flavors except chocolate	½ cup (3 oz.)	135
Chocolate	½ cup (3 oz.)	144
WHISKEY SOUR:		
(Hiram Walker)	3 fl. oz.	177
(National Distillers) *Duet,*		
12½% alcohol	8-fl.-oz. can	256
Mix (Bar-Tender's)	1 serving	70
Mix (Party Tyme)	½-oz. pkg.	50

*Prepared as Package Directs

Food and Description	Measure or Quantity	Calories
WHITEFISH, LAKE:		
Raw, whole	1 lb.	330
Smoked	½ lb.	352
WILD RICE, raw	½ cup	289
WON TON SOUP, canned		
(Mow Sang)	10-oz. can	134

Y

Food and Description	Measure or Quantity	Calories
YAM, raw, whole	1 lb.	394
YEAST:		
Compressed (Fleischmann's)	³/₅-oz. cake	19
Dry (Fleischmann's)	¼ oz.	24
YOGURT:		
Plain:		
(Borden) Swiss style	8-oz. container	131
(Breakstone)	8-oz. container	141
(Dannon)	8-oz. container	136
Apricot:		
(Breakstone)	8-oz. container	220
(Breakstone) *Swiss Parfait*	8-oz. container	249
(Dannon)	8-oz. container	258
Blueberry:		
(Breakstone)	8-oz. container	252
(Breakstone) *Swiss Parfait*	8-oz. container	286
(Dannon)	8-oz. container	258
(Meadow Gold)	8-oz. container	249
(Meadow Gold) Swiss style	8-oz. container	245
(Sanna) *Swiss Miss*	4-oz. container	125
(Sealtest) *Light n' Lively*	8-oz. container	257
(SugarLo)	8-oz. container	117
Boysenberry:		
(Dannon)	8-oz. container	258
(Meadow Gold)	8-oz. container	249
Cherry:		
(Dannon)	8-oz. container	258
(Meadow Gold)	8-oz. container	249
Dark (SugarLo)	8-oz. container	117

*Prepared as Package Directs

Food and Description	Measure or Quantity	Calories
Coffee (Dannon)	8-oz. container	198
Danny (Dannon):		
Cuplet, any flavor	4-oz. container	129
Frozen pop	2½-oz. pop	127
Lemon:		
(Breakstone) *Swiss Parfait*	8-oz. container	254
(Sealtest) *Light n' Lively*	8-oz. container	229
Mandarin orange:		
(Borden) Swiss Style	8-oz. container	227
(Breakstone) *Swiss Parfait*	8-oz. container	263
Peach:		
(Borden) Swiss style	8-oz. container	221
(Breakstone) *Swiss Parfait*	8-oz. container	254
Melba (Breakstone) *Swiss Parfait*	8-oz. container	268
(Meadow Gold)	8-oz. container	249
(Sealtest) *Light n' Lively*	8-oz. container	252
(SugarLo)	8-oz. container	117
Pineapple:		
(Breakstone)	8-oz. container	220
(Meadow Gold)	8-oz. container	249
(Sealtest) *Light n' Lively*	8-oz. container	241
(SugarLo)	8-oz. container	117
Prune whip (Breakstone)	8-oz. container	231
Prune whip (Dannon)	8-oz. container	258
Raspberry:		
(Borden) Swiss style	8-oz. container	236
(Breakstone)	8-oz. container	249
Red (Breakstone) *Swiss Parfait*	8-oz. container	263
(Dannon)	8-oz. container	258
(Meadow Gold) Swiss style	8-oz. container	245
(Sanna) *Swiss Miss*	4-oz. container	125
Red (Sealtest) *Light n' Lively*	8-oz. container	225
(SugarLo)	8-oz. container	118
Strawberry:		
(Borden) Swiss style	8-oz. container	227
(Breakstone)	8-oz. container	225
(Breakstone) *Swiss Parfait*	8-oz. container	259
(Dannon)	8-oz. container	258
(Meadow Gold)	8-oz. container	249
(Meadow Gold) Swiss style	8-oz. container	245
(Sanna) *Swiss Miss*	4-oz. container	125
(Sealtest) *Light n' Lively*	8-oz. container	234

*Prepared as Package Directs

Food and Description	Measure or Quantity	Calories
(SugarLo)	8-oz. container	111
Vanilla:		
(Borden) Swiss style	8-oz. container	235
(Breakstone)	8-oz. container	195
(Dannon)	8-oz. container	198

Z

ZWEIBACK (Nabisco)	1 piece	31

*Prepared as Package Directs